clubfoot connections

clubfoot connections

stories, essays, and poetry from
the clubfoot community

edited by
Betsy Miller

&

Maureen Hoff

Thinking Ink
PRESS

Published by Thinking Ink Press, P.O. Box 1411, Campbell, California 95009
www.ThinkingInkPress.com
First edition, 2023
Paperback edition ISBN 978-1-942480-36-5
Ebook edition ISBN 978-1-942480-37-2

Project Credits
Poetry editor: Keiko O'Leary
Copy editor: Marilyn Horn
Cover design: Streetlight Graphics
Interior format: Liza Olmsted

contents

parenting through the years

walking through life with clubfoot

the story behind
the book

A few years ago, I was brainstorming and sharing ideas for clubfoot books with some clubfoot moms. That might seem a little weird since I'd already written two clubfoot books. *The Parents' Guide to Clubfoot* explains clubfoot and guides the reader through the Ponseti method, which is the recommended treatment. The picture book *Hip, Hop, Hooray for Brooklynn!* celebrates the joy of movement while encouraging brace wear. I believe that different books can offer different kinds of support. I had ideas for several other projects, but before I start on a book about a children's health topic, I talk to parents to find out what they would find helpful. I like to write useful things—it makes me happy and motivates me to know that a book will have a purpose and that reading it might make someone's life a little better.

As I was bouncing around ideas for books, the one that got an enthusiastic response was a clubfoot anthology—a book that would include the personal experiences of people in the clubfoot community. This wouldn't be a book that explains clubfoot treatment; it would be more about the experience of getting through it. I started putting out feelers for who might be interested in writing about their experiences. Kate E. came through with a piece right away, but I wasn't sure about the best method of outreach to get enough additional writers for a book.

As the world moved into the pandemic, Nicole from Clubfoot CARES and I looked into setting up some remote writing events. We thought it might inspire people to write if they hadn't tried before. She contacted the Shut Up & Write! organization about hosting an online group, but it wasn't accepting new writing group leaders at that time. This project went on hold. In the meantime, I focused on creating and publishing a guided journal called *Beyond Boots 'n' Bars*, and a coloring book for kids with characters from the *Hip, Hop, Hooray for Brooklynn!* picture book.

When I saw that Maureen Hoff had written her book *Clubfoot Chronicles*, it was the first book I knew of that was based on the personal experience of a clubfoot mom. I really like her book because it captures her life and inner feelings—almost in real time. Not many people can write that much while they're going through the experience, and if you wait a few years and then try to write about it, most people don't remember the details. It's an amazing snapshot—like a self-created documentary in book form.

I connected with Maureen and we started to get to know each other. She had me as a guest on her Clubfoot Mom podcast, which was fun. Somewhere along the line, I mentioned the clubfoot anthology idea, and she showed a lot of interest. It's similar to what she does on her podcast because it showcases the voices of individuals who have direct experience with clubfoot on a personal level, though she has also had guests on the podcast who are doctors and healthcare workers. I don't even remember asking Maureen if she would be willing to work with me on this project, but I must have because she agreed!

The next thing that happened is I presented the idea for this book to the members of Thinking Ink Press. This is a small publishing company I cofounded and one of the things we publish is clubfoot books. Before we commit to publishing a book, we review the idea as a group. We don't automatically publish every manuscript or book idea that is submitted to our press. In this case, everyone agreed this project was a good idea.

We had a Zoom meeting for Maureen to meet the press members and talk about the project. Because Maureen and I would be developing this book together, we would be coeditors. We figured out pretty early on that Maureen could focus on outreach and inclusion, because she talks to people about clubfoot all the time. Meanwhile, I wrote the call for submissions and would focus on editing the individual pieces in the book, the sequence of pieces in the book, and some of the publishing-related tasks. Maureen and I made a great team because our strengths and skills complement each other so well. We were super happy with all the submissions we received and were able to include all of them in this book. Working on this project has been a joy. I hope you enjoy reading these heartfelt stories from this wonderful collection of writers!

Betsy Miller, Editor

message for clubfoot families

When I was writing *Clubfoot Chronicles*, I was acutely aware that I was speaking from only one clubfoot parent's perspective. I wanted to find a way to get a broader scope of the clubfoot parent experience. When Betsy suggested working on an anthology project, I knew it was the perfect avenue to achieve that goal.

There can be a collective connection through the sharing of individual experiences in a community. That is exactly what this anthology aims to do: to create connection between clubfoot parents. So often when our child is diagnosed with a birth defect and going through treatment, we feel isolated from those around us. Many of us do not see people in our lives going through the same experiences and wonder how they can understand what we are going through. I like to think that by sharing our stories we are allowing people to understand, we are helping people feel less isolated, and we are creating connections between parents.

My sincere hope for this book is that you feel less alone and like you are part of a larger community that truly cares about you. The support and love from those around will make all the difference on your own clubfoot treatment journey.

Maureen Hoff, Editor

starting the clubfoot journey

Receiving a clubfoot diagnosis can be a very intense, emotional experience. As you'll see in these stories, many parents seem to remember this moment vividly. Then as time passes, the memory becomes less emotionally loaded. It's common to need time to process the diagnosis emotionally before being ready to learn more about clubfoot or to talk about it with others.

becoming a mother

Lauren Pruitt

WHEN IS the exact moment someone becomes a mother? Is it when you see those two pink lines on a pregnancy test? Is it when a fresh, wriggly newborn is placed into your arms? Is it when a judge signs papers for an adoption? Maybe it's the first night you tuck in a foster child who's come to live with you, not knowing that one day you'll be their forever home.

For me, the moment that I first felt like a mother was when I went for my first son's anatomy scan. I was 20 weeks pregnant, and this was the big one. This is the one everyone waits for since you can find out the sex of the baby. I had insisted on not knowing the sex until our baby came, but I was still excited to have an ultrasound and see the baby who had started kicking me from inside.

This ultrasound is aptly named the anatomy scan because the purpose is to check baby's anatomy and make sure everything's developing as it should. Brain, heart, spine, kidneys, and everything in between. As the ultrasound technician performed the scan, my husband and I were completely oblivious to the fact that anything could be wrong. There are those moments in life that you don't realize are a before, and this was one of them for us. As the tech got to the limbs, we were mesmerized by those fingers and toes. I remember counting all the toes on one foot and being so excited that all five were there. What more could we ask for?

After the ultrasound, we waited to see the doctor and get confirmation that everything was perfect. That wasn't, of course, what we got. I don't remember the exact conversation, just snippets. Bilateral clubfoot. Probably genetic. You didn't do anything to cause it. Maternal fetal medicine visits. Maybe spina bifida, we'll just check. Don't google any of this.

I felt my heart drop into my stomach. That was the moment when I became a mother. For the first time, the reality of a parent's responsibility came down on me. All the other preparations for baby—setting up the nursery, choosing names, stockpiling diapers—became irrelevant. The full weight of being in charge of this little human being hit me. When this little being arrived, they would need medical care from the beginning. Not only would they need me for the normal baby needs of feeding and changing and comforting, but they'd also need my responsibility and advocacy. They would need my love.

Luckily, clubfoot is an incredibly treatable condition. It's truly a miracle. Babies wear a series of weekly casts that help turn their moldable little feet into the right position. After that, there's a small surgery where the Achilles tendon is snipped since this is shortened and would pull the foot back inward. Finally, there's a brace that babies wear called a "boots and bar" until they're around five years old. At first, they wear it 23 hours a day for three months, but after that it weans down until they eventually just wear the brace only at night.

We're now on the other side, so to speak. My son went through his seven weeks of casts, his months of spending his days in the boots and bar, and now only wearing them at night. In between that time, he learned to walk and run and, much to my chagrin, to climb all manner of dangerous things.

When I first found out that he'd be born with clubfoot, I felt utterly unprepared. How could I possibly be enough? I knew that no matter what, I couldn't take away the pain or discomfort of what he'd go through. For that matter, I'd never be able to shield him from all the other pains and discomforts that life would eventually throw his way. I'd only be able to be with him and love him, which I suppose in the end is what matters most.

the unexpected

Kate E.

ONE HOT AUGUST day when I was eight months pregnant, I was sitting in my older sister's kitchen and explaining—in excruciating detail—how I was trying to determine the optimal timing for when I ought to get the whooping cough vaccine and how antibodies work, and which ones are transmitted through blood versus breast milk. After 20 minutes of my rambling, she looked at me and laughed.

"I'm sorry," she said. "I don't mean to make fun of you. It's just—I know it's always the thing you never expect."

At first, I didn't truly feel the magnitude of the truth in that statement. But just a few weeks later, under the fluorescent lighting of a hospital delivery room, I felt the full weight of it.

Trying to Outsmart Vulnerability

I generally consider myself to be quite an optimistic, hopeful person, and I constantly strive to be open and vulnerable. Up until last year, I had always thought I was both of those things. But from the moment I found out I was pregnant, I googled everything one could ever possibly need to know about how to be the most perfect parent and have the most perfect pregnancy and deliver the most perfectly healthy baby. I was so happy and excited for this new chapter in our lives, and yet the main emotion that seemed to be rising to the surface for me every day was fear.

In an interview with Oprah Winfrey, Brené Brown once said that joy is "the most terrifying, difficult emotion" we can experience. In fact, she even has a term for it—"foreboding joy."

That shocked me to hear. I had always thought of joy as being easy and blissful. But she explained, "What we do in moments of joyfulness is we try to beat vulnerability to the punch." We do this by "rehearsing tragedy" and imagining the worst-case scenario. We try to get ahead of it by preparing for it and figuring out how to strategically avoid it.

And that's exactly what I tried to do. Instead of leaning into the immense joy I should have been experiencing being pregnant, I was looking for all the things that could possibly go wrong and then trying to control and orchestrate life in order to avoid any of those things. I was afraid to be vulnerable.

So, I researched the perfect prenatal vitamins, read articles from various perspectives about the safety of vaccines and ultrasounds, called the doctor whenever I so much as bumped my stomach against a countertop, spent days building my baby shower registry with the highest-rated, nontoxic baby products on the market, and attended 10 weeks' worth of labor preparation classes.

I signed up for every class I could possibly take at the hospital to prepare for my baby's birth and his first few weeks of life. I even attended a course on infant CPR and took copious notes on safety-proofing our home.

I was constantly overwhelmed. I felt like I needed to spend every waking moment figuring out how to avoid my baby being subjected to any harm—and especially how to avoid my being the cause of any. I expected nothing less than perfection of myself, and it was a heavier weight to carry than my growing baby bump.

Kate E.

Labor Day

Despite all my best efforts to control the outcome of my labor, it started just a day before my induction date and lasted 37 hours. The strength of the contractions rendered me nauseated and unable to eat, drink, or sleep. So, after the first 24 hours, though I had spent months preparing for an unmedicated birth, I opted for an epidural.

As I prepared to wait an hour for the anesthesiologist, I closed my eyes as another set of contractions took hold. The nurse assured me that doing so would make it worse and suggested that I keep my eyes open and moan the pain away from myself instead. If only she had known how apropos her advice was for me, the worried woman who had spent 90% of her pregnancy turning into herself and the darkest, most anxious corners of her own mind looking for answers and some semblance of control.

She told me to pick a point on the ceiling and send the pain to it. In my room, there happened to be a pattern with blowing leaves on the ceiling. So, for that next hour, I stared up at them wide-eyed and imagined breathing them away from me like a strong, blustery wind.

Over the next 12 hours, my son's heartbeat started to dip with each strong contraction, and I came very close to needing a C-section. At that point, I was willing to do whatever it took to help him arrive in this world safely, whether or not it had been part of my "perfect plan." However, our doctor tried just one more thing to help relieve any stress on our son. I don't remember exactly what she did, but it worked. Shortly after, I was ready to push.

I had an audience in the delivery room. There was meconium in my amniotic fluid, so they wanted to make sure my son had not inhaled any into his lungs. At that point, unaware of how serious that could have been, I had started to think, "Well, gee, what's one more unexpected issue?!" Between contractions and pushes, I was somehow able to laugh and smile and look people in the eyes as I

scanned the room—my husband, my sister, a few nurses, a neonatologist or two. Everything felt like a slow-motion dream sequence
from a movie—equal parts clear and confusing. It was almost
comical.

As soon as I gave the final push that released our son into the
world, someone (I can't remember who exactly, as it was a bit of a
blur by this point) took him to a little table to examine him and
check his lungs. For a few seconds, things seemed to be okay. I was
anxiously awaiting the moment when my son would finally lay his
crying head upon my chest and find comfort and solace in my
warmth and smell, just like all the babies I'd seen in birthing
videos in our labor preparation classes.

Instead, I saw a neonatologist take my husband aside and
watched his eyes turn from anxious anticipation to a sort of
courageous form of worried. He was trying to hold it together.

"What's wrong?" I asked him.

"Oh nothing, it's not a big deal. He just has a clubfoot," he
replied.

My first thought was that my sister was right. It's always the
thing you never expect.

"What's clubfoot?" I had never even heard of it before.

"His foot is just turned up and inward. They said another
doctor will tell us more later."

I immediately started worrying. My husband lives for physical
activities. He goes spearfishing, rock climbing, hiking, and
camping on a regular basis. Throughout my pregnancy, he had
always told me he intended to take our child with him on all his
excursions out in nature. He wanted to encourage them to have a
taste for adventure.

Suddenly, I wondered what our son would be capable of and
whether he would be able to accompany his dad on all the trips he
had imagined they would take together. I wondered if my son
would always feel different from his peers. I wondered if he'd be in
pain. I wondered if he would endure a lot of suffering.

So, I started asking the doctor and nurses a lot of questions. As I'd practiced throughout my pregnancy, I tried to not sound too anxious out of fear that my concerns might not be taken seriously.

"So, um, will he be able to walk?" I inquired, as the doctor stitched me up.

I honestly don't remember her exact answer. I just don't recall hearing a definitive, "Yes, of course, absolutely." I could understand why a doctor who doesn't specialize in treating clubfoot might not want to make any promises.

"It's actually quite common," she offered. "In fact, there was another baby born here yesterday who has clubfoot."

In a way, that made me feel a bit comforted to know we weren't alone, though I felt for the other baby and their family and still had so many questions. Plus, my sister gently joked later that she wasn't entirely convinced that the doctor hadn't said that just to make me feel better.

Then, after what felt like forever, a nurse walked over to my bedside with our son and started to hand him to me. Before I'd been able to get a good look at his feet, I asked, "Is there any certain way I need to hold him?" I was worried about hurting his little foot.

I will always remember her calm, comforting response that I needed only to hold him just like I would any other baby.

And so, I did hold him like I would any other newborn, which is probably to say with a lot of nervous trepidation. I held him close to my chest and waited for that moment when his screams would subside and he would be calmed upon recognizing my voice and my heartbeat. But that moment didn't come. He continued wailing for quite a while.

In fact, he spent much of the next few days crying, and I kept thinking there was something wrong with me as a mother because I wasn't able to soothe his cries. What I found over the course of his first year of life, however, is that our son just really likes to express himself—and loudly. It has become one of my absolute favorite things about him.

Fear Not the Unexpected

Sadly, when I look back at the first few days of my son's life, I think of how shrouded they were in anxiety and fear. My husband and I felt so overwhelmed with our newfound roles as parents that we didn't even know where to begin with how to learn about clubfoot or its treatment. And for the first time since I had gotten pregnant, I had no desire to consult Google. I didn't know the depth and breadth of the hole I might find myself falling into if I were to open that door. It was all just so unexpected that I didn't quite know how to proceed.

Luckily for us, however, there were a lot of things I had not expected that became reality. For one, our friends and family rallied around us with support and did a lot of research on our behalf. Within just a couple of days, my mom and a friend of ours both came to us with their findings about clubfoot treatment methods and highly rated doctors in our area.

The doctor we ended up choosing was also extremely unexpected. The day I called her office to book an appointment, I recall crying at one point while speaking to the receptionist. Between trying to learn so much about clubfoot in such a short period of time, wanting to get his treatment started as soon as possible, and a whole lot of postpartum hormones coursing through my body, the floodgates had finally opened. She was so understanding and kindly assured me that she would have the doctor give me a call.

Within the hour, my phone rang. The doctor spoke with me for over 30 minutes about what to expect with clubfoot treatment and what our options would be, and she even connected me with other moms who have children with clubfoot. She encouraged me and said that I would be one of those moms supporting new club-foot parents before I knew it.

One of the women she connected me with sent me an unexpected text, which read, "Would you want to talk on the phone right now?" We talked for almost an hour, and I felt so comforted by the end of our conversation.

Within the week, we started treatment with our doctor and her amazing, supportive staff, and we were so surprised at how well our son took to his casts. Before we knew it, six weeks had flown by, and we were already getting him fitted for his boots and bar.

In a way, we had come to love our weekly appointments. It was a special time to bond together, both as a couple and with our son. My mom also joined us at the doctor's office whenever she could, and those are moments I will never forget with her. I never expected that something that seemed so scary in the beginning would turn out to be something that made me feel even more connected to my husband, my mother, and a whole community of parents who had been on similar journeys.

In fact, a week after our son was fitted for his boots and bar, we unexpectedly crossed paths with some fellow patients in our doctor's waiting room. As we were leaving the checkup appointment, there was another couple with a son just about our son's age, and we started chatting.

They were asking about the boots and bar and said their son would be getting fitted for his that day. With hopes of allaying any concerns they might have had, I shared that it had all been going well so far. I said that it was overwhelming at first but already feeling more routine. I asked how old their son was, and his mother replied that he was two months old that day.

As we drove home in the car, I realized that our son would be turning two months old the very next day. Suddenly, I remembered our doctor's reassuring words just after four in the morning when our son was born—another baby had been born with clubfoot just hours before.

When I got home, I found the baby's mom on Facebook through a clubfoot group and sent her a message asking whether she had given birth at the same hospital as I had and what time her son had been born. She replied soon after that, yes, she had delivered him at the same hospital and that her son had been born around four in the afternoon.

So, it was confirmed. They were born 12 hours apart. My son was born nine days late, and hers was born three weeks early. My son was born with a left clubfoot, and hers was born with a right clubfoot. It seemed our paths had been destined to cross.

Later that month, we took some of their first pictures together at a clubfoot holiday party hosted by our doctor's office. The two of them leaned on one another as if they already knew they would be friends. Since then, we've gone on to have play dates together. We talk about the ups and downs of the clubfoot treatment journey, celebrate their progress, and commiserate about how they've both learned to fight getting their boots on at night because they've learned those are an indication that it's time to go to bed. When I'd imagined what my son's birth and first year of life would be like, I had never expected that he and I would make such wonderful friends by bonding over a shared obstacle.

And my son's doctor had been right, too. It was only six months before I became one of the moms to whom she refers other parents who are just beginning the clubfoot journey with their children. I've been on phone calls with worried moms just like me who have just found out their child has clubfoot after an ultrasound appointment and reassured them that they are not alone. I've even had the opportunity to meet a new clubfoot mom and share some of my son's leg warmers to use on her son's casts. I never expected it all to be going by so quickly and to bond with so many other parents in the process.

Every night, my husband runs the nighttime routine of

bathing our son and then putting on his pajamas, stretching his foot, and putting on his boots and bar. It has become their time to bond, and I love watching them together, though the process can be a bit of a challenge at times.

One day, when our son was still getting used to the boots and we were trying to figure out how to pad them to avoid blisters, my husband's brother and sister-in-law were visiting and watching the process.

Our son was crying, and then I broke into tears. I said that it all felt confusing that we were doing something that could seem uncomfortable to him at times, and yet we were doing it because we love him. I shared that I was worried he would associate discomfort with us.

Our sister-in-law gave me a hug and said, "This isn't something you're doing *to* him; it's something you're doing *for* him."

Her words were so comforting. Even my brother-in-law, who can usually be relied upon to crack a joke to ease any tension, got a bit quiet and teary-eyed.

When we first learned our son had clubfoot, I hadn't expected that it would lead to our bonding with our families in such a deep way over a shared love for him. We initially imagined that the clubfoot journey might be one full of nothing but hardship, so I'm endlessly grateful for the abundance of unexpected joys that came out of this experience with our son and loved ones. When I look back, those hidden treasures are the things that I remember most.

Perfectly Himself

Nowadays, those first few months feel quite distant and almost difficult to remember. It often isn't until I see a post in a Facebook group from a concerned parent that I even recall how anxious I was about our son's future and what the path of his treatment would be. I feel so lucky that things have been going well so far, and I attribute so much of that to the amazing doctor and her staff whom we were lucky enough to find, our friends and family who supported us, and so many members of the clubfoot community who have been there to answer our questions and make us feel comforted, especially in the beginning.

One thing I do remember vividly about those early days of parenthood is a friend's comment on the announcement I made on Instagram about our son's birth. He had written, "Oh my goodness, he's perfect!"

And he was right. Clubfoot or not, he is perfect. He is perfectly himself, just as we are all perfectly ourselves.

He is perfectly himself when he expresses his emotions rather vocally and with great passion. He is perfectly himself when he crawls (or walks!) like the wind to escape us whenever it's time for a bath or diaper change. He is perfectly himself when he wakes us up for the fifth time in a night and makes us laugh when we think we may have hit our limit. He is perfectly himself when he flashes his mischievous eyes and grin when we scold him with his full name as he's about to do something he knows he shouldn't. He is perfectly himself when he throws food off of his high chair and bounces his body to the beat of his favorite songs or giggles with his cousins about silly YouTube videos.

He is perfectly himself, and I love who his "self" is more than words can even express.

Open Eyes, Open Heart

Brené Brown says the antidote to foreboding joy is gratitude. And gratitude requires vulnerability. To admit to the universe that I am thankful for the people that matter most to me in all the world is both terrifying and liberating. I'm trying my best to not worry that letting it be known what I'm grateful for will put me at risk of its being taken away. I'm doing all that I can to lean *in* to joy and gratitude and *away* from fear and anxiety.

So, these days, I don't google quite as often, if at all. I've tried to live with my eyes wide open and my heart open even wider. I try my best not to turn inward but, rather, to look around and see all the amazing people we are so lucky to have in our corner—both those we've known for years and become even closer to through this clubfoot experience and those who have become an integral part of our lives in just a year's time.

Whenever our family faces circumstances that feel challenging, I remind myself that sometimes all I need to do is breathe and remember that everything has a way of working out, that we have made it through situations we had doubted whether we could, and that we can do it again and again—together.

I try to soak up each moment with my husband and our son in the same way I wish I had soaked up each moment of my pregnancy. Because I learned that all the planning and the worrying in the world can't keep me from experiencing the unexpected. And sometimes the unexpected is far better than anything I could have ever planned anyway.

Author's Note: I wrote this piece several years ago when my son was a year old, and he recently turned four. He is still expressive and runs from us when it's time to get dressed or brush his teeth. He still charms us out of feeling frustrated with him when he gleefully tests our patience. He still loves to leave a trail of food and toys behind him wherever he goes and loves to sing and dance his way through life. He also loves hiking with his dad and scaling small rock walls on our neighborhood walks. And he loves jumping off things at the playground that are so high it makes other parents gasp with concern.

If things had gone according to what we'd expected, we might gasp, too. But instead, we shout with joy and celebrate the amazing kid he is and how far he has come from that first day we met him in the delivery room and worried whether he would be able to walk. Little did we know he wouldn't just walk; he would also run, hop, skip, jump, wiggle, and dance at every opportunity. My mother, who accompanied us to the majority of his appointments, was watching him play recently and asked, "Which foot is it again?" It has all gone by so quickly. If only we had known. But, then again, if we had, it wouldn't have been quite as beautiful of an adventure.

the phoenix club

Jennifer L. Perrotta

A PREGNANCY at 40 was not planned. Unmarried, unsure, and already a single mother, the timing wasn't great. Before I knew I was pregnant, I had constant pain standing and exercising and decided to get checked out, later to be diagnosed with a femoral hernia. In that same emergency room visit, I received a positive pregnancy test. To further shock my system, I was almost 16 weeks along. I remembered the drinks I had recently had, and the guilt set in and became heavy on my soul. I thought since I'd had my other children in my twenties, the baby train had come and gone from the station. My kids joked that my insides were like the catacombs, a barren space of dust and cobwebs.

Nothing about the pregnancy was easy. My partner was not supportive of the pregnancy at all from the very start, and I was scared to tell my family at first, especially my children. My 11-year-old daughter was happy and excited to add a new member to the family, and she was the only one who showed the "normal" reaction to pregnancy news. But my 16-year-old son and 14-year-old daughter were very upset by the news and my circumstance; they were completely distraught and concerned.

It was an awful feeling to be alone. I went to my first sonogram alone. I remember being scared but also curious about the baby; the gender and just seeing the baby on the screen would make this all more real.

At first, pleasantries were exchanged and I was joyously shown the heartbeat and outline and a few body parts. I was having a boy, but I already felt that in my heart. Then, the ultrasound technician left the room to get the doctor. I was confused, but not entirely worried, just a bit anxious. However, anxiety was the theme of the day. When the doctor arrived and told me the right foot of my baby seemed to be a clubfoot, my heart sank into my stomach. I was trying to process each word she said.

Why was I alone here? That seemed like extra punishment on top of this news. And why had this happened? Was it because I was 40? Was the alcohol to blame? Did my boyfriend and I just have an old egg and sperm? I wanted to blame something, anything. Why did my son have a "curled" foot? I'd had three other children and never experienced this kind of orthopedic problem. Why *this* baby? To add to my anxiety, raging hormones, and utter shock, other ailments needed to be ruled out. It was either idiopathic or an indication of a Pandora's box for this poor baby.

After more testing, I was assured that the foot could be treated, it *was* idiopathic, and everything would be fine—but it was like a death sentence anyway.

As I walked out, I saw happy couples in the waiting room anxiously looking forward to their sonogram and big reveals. I thought, "Their babies are probably not damaged. I did something wrong; my son is damaged."

Not only did I have to tell people I was pregnant, but there was now a huge asterisk as well. "He has a clubfoot, we think just one, but it can be treated. It's going to be turned inward until he gets treatment." Having an asterisk on a pregnancy takes away the joy and excitement really fast. What was already a sticky situation became even more complicated and upsetting.

Results from the amniocentesis at 18 weeks only added a

backpack of bricks on my already weary back and heavy heart. The baby was diagnosed with microdeletion of chromosome 16, group 2A, a complete surprise and no mutation that I carried genetically. It was independent of the clubfoot diagnosis, but with everything stacking up, I was overwhelmed and more deeply concerned for his future and getting to the finish line for the birth.

When I told my dad I was pregnant, it didn't go well because I'm not married and that is one of the biggest sins to a devout Catholic. But when I told him about the baby's clubfoot, that surprisingly went better. Apparently, my grandfather was born with a clubfoot in Italy, and it was repaired there before he came to America as a toddler. He had been deceased for many years, but how did I not know this? It was certainly never talked about during my childhood or as an adult. I felt a rush of relief, yet sadness came over me. I was shocked. So, maybe I didn't "do this" to my baby?! Would my baby be sharing a trait with a grandpa I loved and missed?

Each night at home I poured myself into research and knowledge learning about clubfoot. I wanted to know every possible scenario that would cause this. How could I get this baby help, and what would the outcome be? I was a clubfoot crusader in the night on my computer. I wouldn't give up.

I contacted the clubfoot director at New York University Hospital and had a consult with the clubfoot specialist, while pregnant, to discuss my baby's future treatment. The doctor's calm demeanor and experience made me feel reassured and optimistic that my baby would be in capable hands to help him. It was incredibly overwhelming, though, to understand the treatment journey would be longer than some marriages even last!

At 24 weeks, my baby was diagnosed with intrauterine growth restriction, so I was on pins and needles at every weekly sonogram appointment praying he was growing. Little Leonardo was born at 37 weeks after a difficult pregnancy and a gestational hypertension diagnosis in the third trimester. He was born 5 lbs and 7 oz and 18.9 inches.

I felt like he was the little engine that could. After so much turbulence for him and for me, he was finally born, he was finally here. His right foot was clubbed, just as expected. He was so tiny. At birth he had breathing trouble, so he remained in the NICU for five days, our entire hospital stay. Breathing trouble turned into feeding trouble, and he was connected to machines and tubes around the clock. However, after less than a week, we came home. He was 5 pounds even with his little curly foot. He was just perfect and I couldn't have been happier. My unique Leonardo was here and ready for life's journey. He had risen like the phoenix; all the anxiety, all the physical and mental pain that we'd both endured was now in the past. With his little right clubfoot, Leonardo would now soar like the phoenix.

do you know this baby has clubfeet?

Erica Atha

I HAD JUST GIVEN birth to my son, and my husband and I were in awe of just how perfect he was. I had finally gotten to take my first shower at the hospital. As I was getting out, there was a knock on the door; the hospital's pediatrician was coming in to examine our son. I left the door to the bathroom cracked so I could hear what the doctor was saying. Then I sent my husband to stand with the doctor as he did the exam. To us, our little boy was perfect, but as first-time parents we were nervous about all the "firsts."

As he was doing the exam, I remember the doctor very abruptly asking, "Do you know this baby has clubfoot?"

I proudly exclaimed, "Yes! He was diagnosed at 20 weeks gestation. We have an appointment in January with an orthopedic specialist."

The doctor finished his exam, told us our son looked good, and went on his way.

Once he left, I couldn't help but think, what if I didn't know about my son's diagnosis and this was the way I was finding out? *This* baby that he was referring to was someone's son. My son. I was left feeling like I had been punched in the gut, the same way I felt when I got his diagnosis. This gut punch feeling came from realizing all over again that I would be fighting and advocating for my son every step of his journey.

I know this is something all parents do; we advocate for our kids, but there is something different when advocating for a child born with a birth defect. While he is perfect in every way to me, the reality is that he was born with a birth defect. Our journey will be different than the typical mother/son journey. In some way, I guess I had almost forgotten about his birth defect.

I was so focused on him as a whole and not the treatment of his clubfoot since we had that process figured out. We would meet with the doctor in January. We had a plan, and we would cross that bridge when we got there. Not focusing on his treatment was my way of creating as much of a "normal" pregnancy as possible, even though being pregnant in a global pandemic was far from normal.

Those words from the doctor made me feel like my son was just another baby on his list of babies without his own identity. It catapulted me back to the reality that my son had a birth defect and we would be crossing a lot of bridges along his journey. I wondered how many people learned of their baby's diagnosis from this same type of doctor with a less-than-stellar bedside manner. Would he have taken the time to explain to us my son's bilateral clubfeet, had I said, "No, what is clubfoot?" Or would I have been left to look it up for myself while learning all the other things that come with a newborn?

As someone who works in the medical field, I know just how important a doctor's bedside manner is, especially when delivering a potentially life-changing diagnosis.

I am sure the doctor would have said the same thing had my son been a typical baby. He would have referred to him as *this baby*, and my reaction would have been much different. I don't think I would have had any reaction at all. The clubfoot diagnosis made his words sting. In that moment, I felt like I was the only mom to ever have a baby with clubfoot.

While I knew this was not true, I was not connected with any other moms of clubfoot babies when my son was born. It wasn't until we were almost done with casting that I felt ready to fully dive into the social groups specifically for clubfoot moms like me. I was so overwhelmed with all the things that come with being a new mom that it took me some time to process and really gain my confidence as not only a mom, but the mom of a Clubfoot Warrior.

This wouldn't be the only time I had this feeling of my son being seen just for his birth defect. On another occasion I remember someone seeing my son only for his clubfoot. He was in 23-hour brace wear, and we were on our first family vacation. We made a stop on our way to the beach at a Cracker Barrel shop to stretch our legs. I was holding my son out front, and a couple was sitting in the rocking chairs nearby. I could hear their whispers, and when I turned to them, I saw a look of almost disgust on the woman's face. I did hear some of what they were saying, and it was in reference to someone they knew who had surgery for something similar.

In that moment I felt that all they saw were his boots and bar and not the sweet smiling baby I was holding. Had the interaction gone differently—if they had struck up a conversation about him and his clubfoot—I would've felt different about the whole interaction. It was the stares and whispers that made me feel so alone.

I chose not to speak up in that moment, something I have regretted since that day. We were still in the middle of the pandemic, and there were not many opportunities for my son to be in public with his boots and bar on. I really missed a chance to educate and advocate for him. Until my son can tell his own story, I want his narrative to come from me—not from what strangers think or have learned from other people.

Other times that we went out while he was in 23-hour brace wear, I don't recall anyone staring or whispering around us. If they interacted with us, it was to say how cute he was or something of that nature. It's really too bad that the negative interactions stick out more than the good ones.

Whether you are just starting your clubfoot journey or have been on it for years, know that you are not alone. There is a whole tribe of families who have come before you and will come after you with some of the same experiences and feelings.

a letter to my husband

Casey Murphy

DEAR ETHAN,

The last time I checked, the score was 468-12.

I tell myself that it must be harder for me. I carried him. Surely this is my fault. No one knows why this happens, but that doesn't mean I can let myself off the hook. My job is to protect him, and I got it wrong from the start. When he was born, my anxiety peaked, and all the things that made him cry made me cry. Panic.

But not you. You were so calm and patient. Every week you gently, carefully held onto our swaddled, screaming baby as his foot was stretched and casted. I stood as close as I could, mostly off to the side, crying (but pretending not to) and sometimes shaking. My heart couldn't stand to hear him cry like that, and in the cruel chemistry of those first months postpartum, my body couldn't either. You cleaned us both up. Changed diapers, made dinner, held on tight.

In the blink of an eye, three months passed, and it was time for full time boots and bar. Originally, I thought the boots would be the end of the hard part. But the first time the clubfoot clinic showed us how to put them on, I panicked again. The boots had to be *so* tight. Neil *hated* when they were put on. He cried for 48 straight hours the first time he wore them.

I started to hate the boots, too. Logically, I understood they were important and necessary but emotionally I couldn't get over how terrible they made me feel. They were a clunky, constant reminder of the failure I'd originally felt. I tried to learn how to put them on, but every time it caused me pain, and I imagined it caused Neil pain, too.

I think you understood, so in that same calm and patient way, you took the lead. You started putting them on every day. It got easier over time, but I never asked you to stop. And you never asked me to start.

Now it's 480 days later—give or take—and the score is 468 nights that you've put on the boots, and only 12 for me. I'm bad at it. It makes me nervous, and my lack of confidence is unfamiliar and disappointing. You politely fix my mistakes, but lately I've started to worry that you're disappointed in me, too.

I know it's not really about the boots. I know it's about the pain, fear, and concern that every parent has to process when they learn their baby will be born with a clubfoot. I know it's about the unique teamwork and balance that clubfoot parents have to figure out. And I know that our balance needs some work.

I'm immeasurably grateful to you for never keeping score. But I want you to know that I know it, and I'm working on it every day.

Love,
Casey

the raw reality of a clubfoot mama

Delphine Le Roux

EWEN STARTED his clubfoot journey on May the 4th, 2020, at the age of six weeks because the Covid lockdown had all the clinics canceled for a while. His casting phase started, the weeks were difficult, the days were long. He was constantly crying.

On Mother's Day 2020, I woke up in tears because it was so hard. It was not at all the Mother's Day I had imagined for this year. My friend Liz came to drop off some beautiful flowers for the occasion, which warmed my heart at a moment I needed it the most. What a difficult start of this journey! The nights were terrible; we were reaching a point where we were so tired.

My mother-in-law tried to convince my husband to sleep in the basement for just a night so he could be less tired since he was working. Since she was staying in the guest bedroom next to Ewen's room, she offered to replace Brian for one night in the help he was giving me in going to get Ewen in his bed for his feed and bringing him to me in my bed, and changing his diaper at those times. It did not really work; this is not what we wanted to do.

Although we understood she wanted to help, we wanted to go through this together, suffer together as a team, and support each other through it. My husband did not want to leave me alone. He knew I would break if he did. He was being sturdy so I would not fall apart. He would never leave me on my own while I was struggling, even just for a night to put his own interest or his own sleep first, even though he was working, and I was not. This is not how he loves; he loves deeply and puts his wife's well-being first and foremost. We are just one together, a team that goes through it all together.

We were now at the end of the first week of casting, and so many more were in front of us ... We now had to go back to the hospital to remove the first set of casts and get the next ones put on. Ewen hated when the doctor and nurse were touching his legs. The nurse would remove his casts, sometimes quickly; sometimes it took a lot more time if she couldn't pull easily on the piece of material that is supposed to stick out of the cast to make it easier to remove. Ewen would cry and cry and become all red with his mouth wide open while screaming. Then for a short time, I had the chance to carry him without casts on his legs to get his vitals in a different room (weight, temperature, length) before we came back in the original room to get the new casts put on.

He would curl up against me all soft, which contrasted with the hard casts, and I would enjoy the few minutes of my baby's bare legs. All of this was happening so quickly. It was such a strange feeling to get his bare legs against me without casts. His feet were already looking less crooked. It is crazy the difference one week in casting made. In the cast room, we were back to a round of screams, with Ewen's face all red.

He was so upset the entire time they were putting the casts on that he was not eating anything despite the advice to try to feed him during that time. I tried to feed him afterward, too, but he was too upset. Being so upset would usually wear him out and he would sleep for the next couple of hours. But the sleep was never deep. He would wake up and do little cries or start whining, showing he was in pain or discomfort.

I will remember my entire life that very particular cry. I wish no parent ever had to hear that cry from their baby. Unfortunately, we heard way too much of it. The first night after casting was always brutal. Or should I say, every night during almost the entire casting phase but the first one was particularly more difficult. These were probably the weeks I was the most tired of my entire life.

Ewen spent a lot of time being carried, sleeping on me, and crying during the entire casting phase. Some nights, waking up constantly was just too hard. I had a couple of nights along the way where I would burst into tears in the middle of the night and give Ewen to Brian suddenly after he kept crying while trying to nurse. I would sob like a little girl, sitting up in the bed telling him, "Take him, I can't, I can't anymore. I can't do this; it is too hard. I know I have to be strong, and I can usually be, but this is just too much for me right now." Brian would take Ewen and bounce him to let me collect myself before trying to feed him again.

Those were the nights when even what was supposed to soothe Ewen and calm him down would make him scream even more. While nursing, he had difficulties latching and was getting so upset, which I understood better later when we discovered he had lip and tongue ties.

I felt helpless. If even nursing was not calming him down and making him go back to sleep, what could I do to help him now? My husband was working the next day. I knew this was hard on him, too, but I just couldn't do it. So, I'm glad he was there for me in those hardest times. He would take Ewen away and bounce him to sleep even if it would take forever, just to let me rest. He always helped in the middle of the night, always went to get Ewen to bring him back to me, always took him back to his bed. He dealt with Ewen if he could not fall right back asleep, or brought him back to me if he never fell asleep after a while so he could nurse. Such a good team.

After the tenotomy, it was a really rough patch again for

Ewen. For the entire week, he was crying constantly, in pain, needing to be held or in constant motion. I have a video showing him in our little umbrella stroller, where he starts crying with his very sad and "I'm in pain" cry as soon as I stopped rolling the stroller. I was pushing the little stroller back and forth to calm him down for a long time and he stopped crying as soon as he was moving again. This was our life during this particular week, and for more than only that week actually: CONSTANT CRIES! This was one of the worst weeks, if not the worst. Oh no, the worst week was the one transitioning to boots and bar.

On June 12th, my friend Alex visited us. At that time, I could not take the cries anymore, and thoughts of "throwing my baby in the woods behind my house" were crossing my mind. I remember telling her that, if Ewen was awake, he did not stop crying unless he was in motion. The very next day, I went to a nearby cidery with our best friends. Later, Anchi told me I had said I wanted to throw Ewen in the pond during that visit. I didn't even remember saying this as I was probably just tired and not truly meaning it. I'm sure from an outside point of view, those words are pretty shocking! I would, of course, never have done it. But the fact I could have those thoughts shows how tired I was of those cries, how hard it was to take them in, and how exhausted we were from dealing with all of this.

People talk about mother love, how deeply you love your baby. But honestly, with how much I was taking in, the tiredness and pain from hearing those cries, I did not feel like I had the deep love you are supposed to have for your baby during those times. Or maybe it was because he was born via C-section and the bond was not as strong. I have heard that having a C-section can impact bonding ... No idea if that is true. I really felt like I could not love him fully at this point, even though I was trying. I was attached to him and was there for him no matter what, as my maternal instinct was dictating me to do. The extremely strong love came later; I would say around five months maybe. It is not like I did not love him. I did, but I was not physically and emotionally available to love him as deeply as I could. Maybe I felt some type of weird internal resentment since our life had been shattered with all of this, even though I knew 100% it was not Ewen's fault that he was born with clubfeet.

I guess a lot of moms have those feelings but are ashamed to admit them. I'm not ashamed. There is a lot going on postpartum. Those feelings are normal considering the events. I was doing everything I needed to help Ewen and support him through this, as a mother does. That link was present. I was pushing myself beyond my limits, way past the breaking point, and still going. So, I don't know. It was just too hard to have enough room to love him as much as I thought I should, I guess. The extra love was transformed into strength to power through and make it through all the hard weeks and months. Only when it became easier and that "supernatural" strength was not needed anymore to make it through our days, could the bigger love rise to the surface. I think that is a good way to put it :)

Now onto the transition to boots and bar. The first night was just straight awful, the worst of all, straight torture. Ewen would sleep for 15 to 20 minutes and wake up wailing. Even in our arms where he would usually calm down, he would not. This was torture for all of us. We knew he was in terrible pain but could not stop treatment.

We had been told you can't remove the boots and bar when babies cry. They have to break them in; they will get used to it; it's just gonna be a couple of rough nights. My husband took a few shifts, I took the next ones, and then it was his turn again. I finally decided to finish the night with Ewen sleeping on me. I lay on the bed in the guest room to let Brian sleep, with Ewen against me, thinking, "I will be with you through this entire tough time, my baby. I will not let you down."

I spent hours awake holding him strongly against me while he would cry every 20 minutes. I would nurse him to calm him down here and there, on and off, doze off, cuddle, cries ... It was the hardest night, the longest of all. Twenty-minute increments are really tough.

The next day, my baby was screaming and screaming. Sometimes we could distract him a little. Around 1 p.m. we removed the boots and bar finally for the hour break that was allowed per day. His feet looked terrible, puffy, and bruised, but he seemed pretty happy to be free. His feet were so sensitive after spending eight weeks in casts. Those boots are pretty hard when not broken in. The leather is super hard; everything is harder. Just to put them on is really tough due to the nature of the leather being new, let alone when you are inexperienced.

We never knew if we were fastening the straps too tight or too loose. We had no idea what we were doing basically and felt so scared and at lost. We were mad—mad that nobody trained us better on how to put them on. Especially because, throughout the night, it looked like they slipped. We were saying it's unbelievable that we spend hours getting birthing classes but there is no material available or class to help us navigate through the beginning in boots and bar.

We were beginners; we did not know what we were doing. This entire clubfoot journey felt that way. At first, with the casting phase, we had to relearn everything: how to hold our baby, how to nurse that way, how to change a diaper, etc. And just when we got the hang of it, we switched to boots and bar, where we had to learn everything over again since it is so different. I had three breastfeeding journeys with Ewen: a normal one, a cast one, and a boots and bar one. Each required different positions and tricks and to learn all over again.

This entire clubfoot journey was a hard learning experience, one that we wished we did not have to go through. In the end, the days and nights were long, but the year was short and it all went by very quickly. One thing we knew was that we could only keep going, one day at time, to support him as best as we could.

connecting with others

Having a baby with clubfoot puts parents into a new community for the next four or five years. This can feel similar to the way becoming a parent puts people into a community of other parents. Some people will reach out, and others won't, just like some people happily gravitate toward new moms' groups and others don't.

Most clubfoot treatment happens at home when a child is in a brace, and it's ongoing. This means clubfoot parents go through shared experiences that others who aren't dealing with clubfoot may not understand.

How people connect with others can depend on the opportunities they have and where they live. Some clubfoot clinics help families connect who live in the same area. There are also online clubfoot parent groups that many people join for a while and then leave when they no longer need as much support.

from stigma to sharing

Prina Bagia

WHEN MY HUSBAND and I discovered our baby boy was going to be born with clubfoot, we were shocked, scared, and unsure about the future of our baby. Never having heard of clubfoot, we didn't know if it was going to be a life-threatening disability or if it was treatable. Our doctors did not provide us with resources or information. Also, we were first-time parents and already nervous about how to take care of a baby.

We scoured the internet trying to do our own research to understand the root cause of our baby's impairment and figure out what the course of treatment would be. We learned that the treatment would start as early as the first two weeks of our baby's life. It would start with casting, followed by a minor surgery, and then the correction would be maintained by the boots and bar method. This experience was honestly no different than that of any other clubfoot parents we've talked to or read about. But as new parents, we were extremely concerned with our baby's health, and as individuals of South Asian descent, we had the added layer of stigma that surrounds clubfoot.

Sadly, I was right to be worried about the stigma. We were one of the first families in our community that had a child with clubfoot. We did not know how our community would react to seeing our son casted and then in his boots and bar. Their reaction could have been overwhelming support and wanting to learn about what was going on, or we could have been ostracized for being different because no one would be able to relate to clubfeet. Because we were so unsure, I honestly wanted to hide my baby away from the world. I didn't want him to feel the stares, or to be embarrassed or feel pity, even though at three months old, he wouldn't know what that was, I didn't want him growing up and hearing, "Aw poor thing, look how far you've come." There is NOTHING wrong with my baby, I didn't want it to impact his future.

Another layer to the stigmatization of clubfoot was that we had no external emotional support or outlet for ourselves. My husband and I had to be the experts on the subject. We are not in the medical field, but we had to have all the information ready to share and educate others versus learning the process along the journey. My husband and I felt alienated and burdened by other people's emotions and only had each other to rely on. The emotional and physical toll a delivery takes on parents is unreal, on top of figuring out what to do about clubfeet.

The stigmatization of giving birth and mental health is a huge issue and a topic for another day. People do not share bad birthing stories. When I got pregnant, I only found good or easy birth stories. Only when I started to ask questions and reach out to family and friends did I realize that giving birth is a LOT scarier than the internet makes you believe. Many women don't share their experiences because they are worried about how others will react. Which is why, when it came to my birth story, I openly shared my experience with as many new moms as possible. I gave advice on what to do, what to prepare for, and how to talk to your partner and be open about what is happening.

But I could not take that advice for myself when it came to my baby's clubfeet. I was so worried about how people would react and treat him that, during serial casting, I gave in to the stigma and didn't share anything related to his feet, and instead putting on a happy face.

I decided to share my baby's clubfoot journey after he had his tenotomy surgery. At this point, we wouldn't be able to hide what he was going through, and the world would now see his feet in the boots and bar.

My motivation unfortunately was to mitigate the "bad press" that comes from this sort of physical appearance. I want to say that I was noble and decided to share the news with the world so I could seek support, meet more parents, share my stories, and increase the awareness of clubfoot. But that's not the truth. I was worried about how my friends and family would pity me, my husband, and my son. They would say things behind our backs or say how "sad" it was or give us condescending praise for how well we were doing.

In our community, like many others, if anyone looks, acts, or thinks differently, they are automatically ostracized and talked about. And it does not just affect one person, but the entire family they are a part of. I didn't want that. I didn't want my parents to feel bad because people were saying bad things about us. I didn't want my siblings to have to defend us because of how scary clubfoot looked. I just wanted a "normal" baby and to blend in with the crowd.

After realizing my motivations for why I wanted to share our stories, I felt ashamed. Why did I care so much about what my community thought versus actually sharing my experience and helping others? Then I realized that my son, my husband, and I were never going to be "regular, normal" people. We were tasked with raising the awareness. We were tasked with bringing a voice to others in our community and speaking up. At the time, it was exhausting and scary to take on that burden, but having gone through it all, we are better for it.

Whenever we meet anyone and their eyes go directly to my son's boots and bar, I openly share his condition. I want people to understand what he has and that this is more common than a cleft lip or allergies, and that this is nothing deadly or anything that will impair his future. I share stories on his progress. I share images of what his feet looked like before and what they look like now. I share the fact that his feet are fixed and he's physically thriving. He's starting to crawl; he's learning how to swim; he's trying to stand; he sits up by himself—all before the age of six months! I want to remove the stigma that clubfoot is a lifelong impediment that will ruin any child's life.

There are a lot of people out there who think that asking a question is rude or shameful, but it's the exact opposite. Asking questions shows you care and want to learn. What's rude is staring at someone's impairment, talking behind their backs, or faking praise.

I want to share my story with the world, to show everyone that it's okay to be worried and scared for your child, but you shouldn't be worried or scared about what others think. As a parent, you do the best you can with the knowledge you have to take care of your baby, and no one knows your baby better than you do.

And as scary as it may seem, you are not alone. You can connect with and talk to others who have gone through this journey every day to get the emotional support you need. And as a parent of a clubfoot cutie, we spread the word as much as we can to bring that awareness forward.

online clubfoot
community with heart

Tiffany Johnson

TO SAY I got sucked into a searching spiral after our son's clubfoot diagnosis is a bit of an understatement. It nearly consumed me. The afternoon of our anatomy ultrasound looked something like this:

Opens search bar and types:

- "What is clubfoot?"
- "What causes clubfoot?"
- "Does clubfoot point to an underlying condition?"

Once I'd sufficiently pored over information, I moved from text to visuals. I needed to know what to expect when we first saw our beautiful baby boy and he started treatment.

Switches to the images section of the search bar:

- "Clubfoot pictures"
- "Babies with clubfoot"
- "Clubfoot casts"

After hours of research, I was left feeling somewhat informed and completely overwhelmed.

The internet may have given me an introductory understanding of our son's clubfoot diagnosis, but it didn't give me much peace of mind. I kept replaying moments from our appointment earlier that day: everything was going so well until my husband and I noticed the ultrasound technician focusing rather intently on our son's foot. After finishing up, the tech said the doctor would be in shortly. The doctor reviewed the images, took another look, and referred us to a specialist to follow up on our son's suspected right clubfoot.

That was that.

We'd planned to go out after our appointment—ultrasound pictures in hand—to celebrate our growing baby. Instead, we skipped lunch and drove home in near silence. I spent most of the drive staring at the printout of my sweet son's right (club)foot.

There's no history of clubfoot in our family that we know of. I didn't have any friends who'd experienced this with their babies. I wasn't sure who or where to turn to for support. There was also mention of additional ultrasounds, a fetal echocardiogram, an MRI, and/or an amniocentesis as a follow-up, and it was all a lot to process.

I felt alone.

That's when I hopped on Facebook and joined a clubfoot support group. If I didn't find it helpful, I'd leave. No biggie. I figured I'd scroll through a few posts to get some insider tips from parents and caregivers who'd been on this journey. Maybe find some information an internet search wouldn't uncover.

To my surprise, the clubfoot group felt more like an online community of friends than a virtual gathering of strangers. There were so many messages of encouragement and support. I was blown away by the openness, kindness, and helpfulness displayed in the group.

I was immediately comforted.

Here's a glimpse into the valuable insight and knowledge shared in this online community:

- Clubfoot doctor recommendations by area. We found the perfect doctor for our son by reading dozens of glowing reviews from real parents and caregivers on the page.
- Lists of items that may be useful during treatment. We stocked up on no-rinse baby wash for the casting phase, moleskin, and snap-up rompers for bracing with boots and bar.
- Sentimental suggestions like documenting your child's clubfoot journey and grabbing an infant plaster casting kit to capture their "super foot" before treatment as a keepsake, both of which we did.
- Before and after pictures documenting the amazing transformation your baby's foot goes through during treatment.
- Perfect positions for nursing a newborn in casts and an infant in boots and bar.
- An unfiltered look into the world of clubfoot treatment—from the occasional sleepless night to the joy and awe of seeing your baby's corrected foot.
- Example messaging for baby shower invitations, including clothing suggestions to accommodate casts and/or boots and bar.
- Firsthand experiences with specific car seats and carriers and how well they work with boots and bar.
- Tips for potty training a child in a brace, as well as safely making the transition from a crib to a toddler bed.
- Reassurance that kids can indeed roll, crawl, walk, and hop in boots and bar. Watching videos of happy kids

accommodating the brace made it seem less intimidating.

- Encouraging messages from families of kids who finished treatment. Seeing former clubfoot babes turned tennis stars, long-distance runners, and elegant dancers helped keep things in perspective. It was a refreshing reminder that, one day, this will all be behind them.

I appreciated the realness and rawness of the group as well. Scrolling through, stories about relapses and pictures of blisters, slipped casts, and bruises popped up. No one wants their child to experience setbacks during treatment. It was helpful to see, though, that even with unexpected obstacles along the way, these kids thrive. On top of that, these images often included tips on what to look for before a little problem like a red mark becomes a bigger problem like a pressure sore. We knew what to watch out for and when to reach out to our doctor.

That alone is invaluable information.

I remember asking the group about babies rolling back to tummy relatively early with boots and bar on because our son kept waking himself up at night trying out his new skill. It seemed like the brace gave him the leverage to roll over before he was ready to. Though I felt for other families experiencing sleepless nights, it was reassuring to hear that more restful sleep should come once a braced babe figures out this whole rolling thing.

I was thankful to have found my clubfoot community that I could turn to any time of night.

Sure, there've been some challenges along our son's clubfoot journey. But, true to his character, he's powered through every step of treatment with a smile on his face. He's a shining light in our lives and inspires us every day. Just as we'd encouragingly read in countless posts in the group, having a clubfoot has never held him back. He's our rock star.

clubfoot community

Abby Skinner

THE DAY HAD FINALLY COME—THE day my son's last set of casts would finally be taken off and he would receive his boots and bar. My son, husband, and myself were in the hallway outside the casting room waiting for our turn with the doctor when we began to hear the cries of a newborn baby. I was holding my precious baby boy and I could not help but think about how far we had come in our clubfoot journey since my son's first appointment with the orthopedic doctor at two weeks old. There had been 11 sets of casts, two slipped casts, blisters, bruises, and the tenotomy surgery.

I was constantly writing down questions for the next time we would see the doctor. Throughout the casting process, there were days where all I could do was snuggle my baby to help him feel better. I cannot imagine how he felt having casts on and not being able to move his legs and feet the way he wanted to. I began to worry about him constantly and always felt judged when we would go out in public and people saw his casts.

I started feeling guilty and alone even though I was surrounded by family and friends giving us encouragement and support. Depression took over without me even realizing it. Yes, I would smile and try to say the right things when people asked questions about my son's feet, but I was struggling with feelings and emotions that I still cannot put into words. My son eventually got used to the casts and amazed me with each new milestone he met. I'll be honest—he handled the whole treatment process better than I did. Clubfoot babies have unbelievable strength and resilience.

Now, the casting room was open. It was almost time for us to see the doctor, so I settled into the room. My husband went to fill out some paperwork at the front desk, and that is when I saw her. I saw the mother of the baby who was crying. He was wearing his first set of casts. The mom was sitting on the other side of the room rocking her baby and soothing him before they left to go home. I could not help but notice that she was crying and she was alone at the appointment with her baby.

I was not going to say anything to her at first because I did not want to make her feel uncomfortable or embarrassed, but then I thought to myself that I wished someone was there at our first appointment to offer some advice or kind words. I spoke up and told her that it does get better with time and the treatment will all be worth it in the end.

She wiped her tears and told me thank you. She walked over and started asking me questions—questions that I actually had the answers to since we had been through many weeks of treatment already. I made sure to tell her that clubfoot babies' journeys can be different from one another, but we are all working toward the same goal. I gave her some advice and some tips and tricks I had learned along the way. Before she left, I told her that she was a wonderful mom for being strong for her baby and we wished each other well.

We finished with the doctor and were on our way home. I sat in the back seat with my baby and watched him sleep soundly wearing his new boots and bar. The other clubfoot mom was on my mind. I felt so thankful I was able to have a conversation with her, offer her some hope, and see her begin her own clubfoot journey with her baby boy. The fact that I helped another mom opened my eyes to the meaning behind the saying "it takes a village." I looked for clubfoot support groups on social media and found one on Facebook that I immediately joined.

Reading about other clubfoot babies and their families' journeys made my feelings of loneliness melt away. I continued reading different posts and comments of clubfoot moms and families giving advice, compliments, and words of kindness to one another. I found a clubfoot community—a place where parents and loved ones from all over the world shared my fears, worries, hurdles, and questions. Clubfoot babies and their caregivers are some of the strongest people I have ever known. Yes, there is treatment and clubfoot can improve over time, but we need each other to get through the bad days *and* good days.

That moment was a turning point for me in the best way possible. It made me realize how blessed I am to be among a population of moms, dads, and family members who are proactive in getting the treatment their child needs and do everything they can to make sure that their child can be successful in the future. This whole experience has taught me what it really means to be a mom and has given me the most amazing relationship with my son. He is the happiest little boy and has changed my life for the better. I am forever grateful for my clubfoot cutie and everything my family has learned and overcome along the way.

coleman's clubfoot journey

Jessica Norris

I CAN REMEMBER it like it was yesterday. The day was November 22, 2021. I had just left my 20-week prenatal appointment and anatomy scan. I can still remember the feeling when my OB told me that Coleman appeared to have clubfoot. At first, I didn't cry. I just sort of held my breath and looked at my husband with fear in my eyes and saw him looking back with the same expression.

This was the first time I had even heard of clubfoot, much less that it was treatable. Of course, every thought started running through my mind. "Will my son ever be able to walk?" "What's the treatment like?" "Will he be in pain?"

After we left the appointment and got into the car, I burst into tears. My doctor had given me assurance that everything would be fine. This was just a bump in the road and everything was going to be okay. Yet I couldn't stop blaming myself for the diagnosis. What could I have done to prevent this? The emotions were overwhelming on top of all the pregnancy hormones. I felt like a complete failure to my son.

Since I was only halfway through the pregnancy, I decided to dive into researching everything I could to learn about clubfoot. That's when I came across more resources than I ever would've realized. I became infatuated by clubfoot content and the community of parents who rally behind their kids to support their treatment. I became stronger because of the clubfoot community, and I felt prepared to take on the challenge of treatment.

Coleman was born on March 31, 2022, with bilateral club-foot. A week after his birth was his first orthopedic appointment at Children's of Alabama where he received his first set of casts. His physician was thorough in explaining the clubfoot treatment process and how each cast was set in particular forms to correct the feet. As we were leaving Coleman's first appointment, we saw another little boy with full leg casts in the waiting room. I couldn't help myself and I ran over to his mom. The child was going to his orthopedic appointment to remove his last set of casts, and it gave me so much hope that Coleman would be in that same position within time.

Casting was an adventure, but nothing that wasn't unman-ageable. Diaper changes were challenging, and not being able to dress our little boy in cute footed pajamas was disappointing, but those were things that we could easily learn to accept. Coleman's care was our greatest concern and, for the most part, he handled the casts with ease. He slept fine with them. He honestly didn't know the difference since it was all he really knew. I'm a huge advocate for starting the casting as early as possible for this specific reason.

However, I would be naïve to not mention that there were definitely hard times as well. Aside from the physical trials, we faced many emotional tests. Going out in public with Coleman's full leg casts was bound to turn heads. I would get looks of concern and could almost hear what the other person was think-ing: "Did she break her son's legs?"

I would notice the confusion on people's faces and immedi-ately speak up to tell them it was okay to ask about his condition. Even though it felt like I was constantly repeating the same lines to describe clubfoot, every time I did so felt like a sense of peace. Somehow it felt comforting to share his story and assure people that clubfoot is treatable. In fact, the more I shared about Coleman's clubfoot journey, the more people would share about someone they knew who went through the same thing.

Coleman stayed in casts for five weeks before moving to boots and bar. I didn't want to rush the process, but I will be honest: there was definitely a countdown app on my phone with remaining days until he would be out of casts. It was starting to get into the heat of early summer in Alabama. It was getting harder to keep Coleman cool with the thick casts he was wearing. On May 23, 2022, Coleman received his first pair of boots and bar.

Coleman stayed in 23-hour boots and bar wear for about four months before reducing wear-time to only nights and naps. He will continue wearing his boots and bar at nights and naps until he's reached a year old. Then his doctor will reevaluate to see if he can reduce wearing them to nighttime only. Being free from casts has allowed Coleman to finally enjoy activities like bath time and swimming.

He's also hitting milestones that many of his nonclubfoot friends are reaching. With his boots and bar, he's still been able to learn to roll over and is attempting to crawl at six months old. My husband and I champion Coleman and constantly use words of affirmation to encourage him to stay strong. While he's still too little to truly understand the extent of what he went through and what he continues to endure, I know there's going to be a day when he asks me about his shoes. That's when I feel like the true tests will come.

Through the clubfoot community, I've learned many tips from other parents on how to approach this when the time comes. For now, we just take things day by day. It's definitely not an easy journey, but knowing that there's others out there in the same position helps me not feel alone.

So, thank you to the community of parents who spoke out about the Ponseti method to push it as the standard, thank you to the parents who are vocal about their child's journey to better prepare others who face the same challenge, and thank you to those who spend countless hours bringing together this clubfoot community. If I could go back to that day at my 20-week anatomy scan, I'd tell my scared pregnant self that everything is going to be okay. Your son will be strong and resilient, and he will be running circles around any obstacle he faces. You are not alone: you got this, Momma.

from anger to advocacy

Nicole Bytnerowicz

WHEN I STARTED my clubfoot journey seven and a half years ago, I never could have imagined that I was going to start a nonprofit dedicated to clubfoot. In fact, when my son was diagnosed at the 20-week ultrasound, I stuck my head so far into the ground that I refused to even join support groups on Facebook. Joining a support group would be me admitting that my son had a problem. I kept my head down and kept telling myself, "It'll be a quick fix, and he won't even remember it one day! A blip in my life as a mom." I could accept that he would be born different, but I didn't need to accept that this was part of my identity as a mother. I was not a clubfoot mom. I was a mom with a child who had clubfoot.

I only ended up joining the Facebook groups when I thought my son had completed his castings, as a way to celebrate being "out of the woods." I then had the wind knocked out of me when more seasoned clubfoot parents informed me that my son's case was complex. I looked back on my short journey and thought of how "easy" everyone said it would be, so I never bothered researching potential red flags or what was "proper treatment." I assumed my doctor would handle everything and it would be a "quick fix."

So, when my son's treatment wasn't as straightforward as expected and my doctor suggested an invasive surgery to fix it, I searched for a second opinion and transferred care to Iowa where the Ponseti method had been developed. Once the dust settled and he had finished being retreated, my acceptance regressed to anger. I was angry that I had to travel so far from home when my son should have received topnotch care with his original doctor. I was angry that I hadn't educated myself properly. I was angry that the resources weren't easy to access. But then something started shifting in me. My anger lit a fire in me that I didn't know I had until I became a mom. I realized I wasn't alone, and that my son's situation mirrored those of thousands of other children. I realized my son's case turned out the way it did because I wasn't fully educated on clubfoot and the proper treatment method, but that I could somehow fix that problem.

When I posed questions in the Facebook groups, I would be redirected to previous posts with the same questions and answers. Parents were constantly posting the same questions and receiving the same answers from other parents. There was so much redundancy. And when looking for more information online, I found myself spending hours looking all over the internet for pieces of it. The only clubfoot-dedicated nonprofits I could find serviced other countries, and they focused more on treating kids than educating their caregivers. None of them were focused specifically on US demographics.

I decided I didn't want more families to face what we had faced. I, along with three other moms, decided to start a nonprofit that focused on educating and empowering families to advocate for their children's clubfoot care. We created a website that was a culmination of years of clubfoot parent experience, and helped create a community that I had initially denied wanting to be a part of.

Remember those other clubfoot nonprofits I mentioned? Their cofounders are some of the most inspiring humans I've ever

met. I quickly discovered that starting a nonprofit is insanely difficult. I had just left my full-time job when we cofounded it in
November 2016, and found myself working full-time hours again
just to get it off the ground. Except this time, I was unpaid, so it
was truly a labor of love. From incorporating Clubfoot CARES,
to finding pro bono expertise to get our tax exemption status, it
took hundreds of emails and phone calls. When we got our federal
tax exemptions status, we cried. Every dollar that was donated
ended up having a direct purpose to operating our nonprofit. We
were able to get our website built and information logged.

A few years later when a parent-operated initiative for
receiving and redistributing donated boots needed to find a new
home, we were able to adopt it at Clubfoot CARES and operate it
with amazing volunteers. Our digital imprint spans over 75 countries, supports a community of nearly 6,000 people (and growing!), and has helped hundreds of families get access to free boots
to allow their care to continue unrestricted by the financial
restraints they often face when getting medical care. We are the
US representative for a global clubfoot organization that was also
started by parents, and we continue to partner with larger, more
established nonprofits that are working to make the world a better
place.

I have spent thousands of hours talking about my son, our
journey, this nonprofit, and all things clubfoot over the last seven
years. I have listened to countless parents crying on the phone. I
have cried on the phone to countless parents. Years of tears, frustration, as well as happiness and triumph. And every time I want
to throw in the towel and give up, I get a simple "thank you" from
a parent and it pushes me to continue on. Clubfoot isn't going
away, and I hope neither will Clubfoot CARES.

Now, I'm here from the "other side." My son is seven years
old, but his clubfoot will always be a part of him. He knows he
has to do nightly stretches to prevent relapse, even if he's not
super fond of them. But he's okay. He's thriving. He's running,

jumping, and playing sports. He plays with his friends and he lives a normal life. He's funny, strong, and an amazing human being that I'm proud of daily.

So here is what I have to say to you parents: your kid will be stronger than many other kids. They will know what it feels like to face challenges. They will feel a lot of pain, but they will be okay. They will struggle to do tummy time, but they will work around it. They will become innovative in how they use their legs, and it'll surprise you. And they will bang the crap out of your hardwood floors, and probably various parts of your body if you're holding them when they get excited, and the bruises all over your body will be a reminder of that.

And guess what about you? YOU will be stronger than you ever thought possible. You will see your child in pain, and you will force yourself to hold it together for them. You will hold their little hands through the castings, and you will cuddle them so hard after their tenotomy. You will have a new appreciation for their new feet, and it'll inspire you to sign your kid up for ballet and soccer. It may even motivate you to use your own feet more. You'll kiss their toes and you'll love your baby just as much as if they were born with straight feet. You may even love them a little bit more because you had to fight for them.

Every trip to the doctor is you advocating for them, so give yourself grace and a tight hug. I know what you're feeling right now. You're feeling scared. You're feeling anger, maybe. You're grieving the future you thought you'd have. And that's okay. Soon enough you'll be in my position, forgetting why you even worried in the first place. Oh, and start telling people about your kid's clubfoot. You'll be surprised how many people tell you they had it when they were little! The best thing that has come from this whole experience is that you will forever be a part of this elite group of parents who will welcome you and love you and help you, no matter what.

parenting
through the years

For most parents, the focus on their child's clubfoot treatment occurs mainly in infancy and early childhood. As their child stops wearing a brace, life gets busy, and different things become important in day-to-day life.

For some kids, clubfoot requires addition treatment after age five. This additional treatment is less likely to be needed if a child is treated with the Ponseti method. That said, some kids have residual clubfoot or clubfoot together with another health condition, which might mean that a child has a foot surgery such as a tendon transfer.

Most people don't need to travel thousands of miles for clubfoot treatment, but in some of these compelling stories, that's exactly what these families did.

In this section, several parents wrote about their experiences, and you can find corresponding perspectives from their children in the next section, "Walking Through Life with Clubfoot," on page 91.

owen's clubfoot journey

Marlene Parry

OUR SWEET BABY Owen was born with bilateral congenital talipes equinovarus (clubfoot).

Clubfoot is a deformity in which an infant's foot is turned inward and the bottom of the foot faces sideways or upward. Clubfoot affects 1 in 1,000 babies worldwide. I don't write this to scare anyone, especially someone going through this with their clubfoot cuties, but to know that your sweet baby and you WILL get through it. It WILL get easier. It is hard, there's no denying that, but you and your baby are stronger than you ever knew!

Because of Covid, I went to my 18-week anatomy ultrasound alone. The doctor told me that our baby's right foot was club and potentially his left. I needed to have another more in-depth ultrasound as the clubfoot deformity can be a characteristic of many other disorders and syndromes. I honestly had no idea what clubfoot was or what it even meant. I had no idea what to expect or if my baby would be okay.

The doctor showed me a picture of a baby's foot twisted inward and upward. I felt so overwhelmed, confused, and beyond sad that my baby could be in pain. I phoned Joe and then my mom to let them know what I had learned. I was devastated. I cried with my mind racing the whole way home from London. I was terrified at the thought that this could be a sign of something worse for our baby.

At the next ultrasound, they did a very thorough scan of all his body parts and took a ton of measurements ultimately ruling out, to the best of their ability, any other issues. They did confirm that he had bilateral clubfoot (meaning in both feet), but that the clubfeet were isolated and not related to any other issues that could be determined in utero. The doctors reassured me that it was treatable, but it would be a long process of casting, surgery, and bracing.

One of the most incredible and magical moments in my life was seeing Owen for the very first time. My doctor bouncing him up and down right beside me, I saw the most beautiful, pudgy, roly-poly boy. He was absolutely perfect, and I was so in love. I never even noticed his feet. The first time I unwrapped him from his blanket I looked at his feet, and yes, his feet were crooked, but to me they were perfect.

The first eight days with him were full of emotions, love, and bonding as Owen stayed in the NICU. We weren't home long before we began his clubfoot journey.

At 20 days old, Owen started his clubfoot treatment. I wanted to remember his feet just as they were. I loved those imperfect feet. They curved where the arch of his foot would have been and at an unnatural upward position, but all I saw was perfection. When he pulled his legs in, his feet would tuck right up to his bum and his legs would make a heart shape.

As odd as it sounds, I didn't want to go and get them fixed. Yes, I understood that he couldn't walk with his feet like this, so I knew we had to get them fixed and starting treatment as soon as possible was the best option. At the first appointment with our pediatric orthopedic surgeon in London, he manipulated Owen's feet into a more "normal" position and casted both legs from his toes to his upper thigh. This first casting, along with all those that followed, I stood next to Owen and watched him scream and cry cries I had never heard before and turn a tomato shade of red.

I felt so helpless, unable to console him, that I broke down, too. He was so uncomfortable, and the casts were heavy, wet, and cold. The drive home was awful and sleep that night was nonexistent. The first night after each casting was by far the worst. I'd rock him, bounce him, try to warm the tips of his toes that were cold from the casts that took 24 hours to dry, but the crying would stop for only small amounts of sleep at a time.

It was like he was begging us to remove the heavy weight on his legs. He was so fussy from gas and unable to move or bend his legs to help move the gas through. That night I cried with him, too, hoping it would all be over soon. Having a baby in casts was hard; we couldn't even bathe him. If he got poop on his casts, I just had to wipe them the best I could. I couldn't wear him in a carrier, he couldn't wear pants or footed pajamas, he was awkward to hold in some positions, and he was hot in those casts.

As each day came, it did get easier. Owen would get used to the new position of his feet, the cast was dry and no longer cold or as heavy. We went back to London weekly to have the casts removed, feet stretched further, and new casts put on where we would repeat the same screams and cries, the same shade of red, the long drive home and sleepless nights. He ended up developing a large umbilical hernia due to the pressure on his stomach muscles from the weight of the casts. During these weeks we struggled, but we survived.

At six-and-a-half weeks old, Owen's fourth set of casts were removed, and his feet were in a "normal enough" position that he then had surgery on each of his feet. Attending all the appointments alone was hard, but the Achilles tenotomy surgeries were beyond difficult. I had the choice to be with Owen during the surgeries and didn't want him to be alone, so I rubbed his head and he held my finger as he incessantly screamed and cried during both procedures. It was so difficult to watch that I couldn't for the second foot. I kept my eyes on Owen's face as I continued to do whatever I could to console him. After each surgery, he was recasted. This set of casts stayed on for three weeks while the tendon that was cut during surgery reattached itself.

On June 17th, Owen got his final set of casts off. We immediately went to an orthotic clinic where he was fitted for his boots and bar. I had been so looking forward to the braces as another step closer to correction. I convinced myself that everything would be better when we were done with casts, but that did not turn out to be the case. The braces are heavy, too, and confining, and something I hadn't even considered was how sensitive his feet would be.

His feet had been in casts and not touched for seven weeks. Each time his foot slipped or we took a break (he got one hour every day), it was dreadful putting them back on. He screamed and cried. He consistently had blisters in new places. But, just as the casting phase got easier, the boots and bar did, too. He had to wear them for 23 hours a day until September 30th, when we got the okay to go to naptime and bedtime wear.

In March, Owen's surgeon was impressed with the flexibility in his feet and eliminated the need for naptime wear. Owen is now only wearing his boots and bar for 12 hours through the night, which will continue until he's over four years old! He is currently on his fourth set of boots and is frequently seen by his pediatric orthopedic surgeon and his orthotist in London. Getting them on most of the time is a bit of a wrestle, but he truly is so patient, and you'd never know all he's gone through with his absolutely hilarious personality!

Navigating each stage has been extremely hard, and I can't even begin to fathom the strength it has taken Owen to go through all of this. I am in awe of Owen, and forever will be, for all his fight, strength, and resilience.

dad saves the day

Chidiogo Obiesie

MY HUSBAND HAS ALWAYS BEEN a hands-on father and husband, and the way he carries about his fatherly duty is admirable. Even though he is a father of our four children, he makes sure he is directly involved in the affairs surrounding his family. One remarkable thing about my husband is the way he took good care of our daughter, Tobe, while she was ill.

Tobe is our seven-year-old daughter who was born with congenital clubfoot. She's a very smart and vibrant child. Even with the situation surrounding her birth and early childhood, Tobe still remained cheerful and energetic.

When Tobe and her twin sister were born, my husband and I never imagined that one of our daughters would be born with a congenital clubfoot. In fact, we had never heard of it until Tobe's birth. You could imagine how clueless and sad we felt after we discovered the condition. Regardless, my husband and I were still grateful for the gift of our daughters. My husband and I loved our girls and both he and I decided there and then to put in all efforts just to make sure Tobe was fine, notwithstanding the time and resources it might cost us.

The first step my husband took was to read about the condition—congenital clubfoot. He spent many days surfing the internet, reading articles and watching videos about it. The doctors were also kind, and they took the time to educate us about what the condition was all about. Deep down, my husband and I knew it was going to be a very long journey.

At one point, my husband became discouraged. He thought the condition was incurable and his daughter might not be able to walk well. He had no prior knowledge of the condition and could not say for sure if the condition had a cure. He was really on the verge of giving up until a miracle happened.

The miracle was a man whose son had a similar issue, although his was mild compared to that of Tobe. The man assured my husband that the condition could be treated just like his son's.

At last! There was hope for my husband.

He picked himself up again and continued researching the condition. All the while, I was at the hospital. I had to stay longer in the hospital since I gave birth to my twins with a C-section. We really never expected things to turn out the way they did. I would cry and cry. It was my husband who consoled me and asked me to stay strong.

Tobe commenced her clubfoot treatment at five days old. Both her father and I had mixed feelings about this. We were scared of the unknown since we had never had such an experience before. At the same time, we hoped that our daughter would get better as soon as possible. We thought that the treatment would last for a short period until the doctor told us that the treatment would last for three to four years. My husband and I didn't like the sound of that; we were overwhelmed. What it meant was that Tobe's legs would take a lot of time to be corrected. Both of us were expected to make sure she wore her correction shoes every night, until the treatment gradually ended.

At this point, my husband knew he had to be there for his daughter.

On the first day of the cast, I was not emotionally or physically strong enough to join in the casting room, so my husband took Tobe on his own.

All through the day after the casts, my husband carried Tobe. She would cry and cry. My husband, in a bid to calm Tobe down, discovered she remained calm while he played music: one particular song was very soothing. Once the music was on, Tobe would be calm. That particular song later became our after-cast song. My husband was the only dad who accompanied his wife to the hospital. Whenever Tobe has an appointment with the doctor, he would drive both Tobe and me to the hospital. He would also accompany us to see the doctor. My husband was a great support system; eventually I became stronger.

The Orthopedic Hospital

"There is a cut on that boy's leg!" I shouted.

A young boy was bleeding. It was our second day in another hospital. The first hospital referred us to this orthopedic hospital so that Tobe could be fitted for braces. When my husband and I got here, the doctor insisted that Tobe's legs had not been corrected. They had to begin another round of treatment.

On the second day, when my husband and I took Tobe for her treatment, the assistants were supposed to remove the casts off Tobe's legs. They were making use of a noisy machine to remove the casts. The children would cry and cry as the cast removal was ongoing. The children would struggle, and during that process a child's leg got cut.

My husband called my attention. He saw how scary it was. He didn't want the doctor to use the machine on Tobe's leg, so my husband quickly rushed out to get a surgical blade. Gently, he removed the casts off Tobe's legs with the surgical blade. The cast had to be wet so that it could be removed gently. I had a sachet of water with me, so we wet the cast with the water, and he continued.

It took my husband over an hour to remove the casts from his bilateral clubfoot girl, as against the ten minutes removal with the scary machine. My husband took his time to remove the casts off Tobe's legs. Then he took her to the casting room so that the doctor could assess her.

That was how Superhero Dad saved his daughter.

He didn't want his daughter to go through the traumatic experience of the noisy machine. It makes a loud noise, and a lot of children cry profusely whenever it is used on them. My husband didn't want that for Tobe, so he continued removing the cast by himself throughout the casting period in that hospital.

Genu Recurvatum

Tobe continued to grow, although she still couldn't walk well except with her braces. She was in her third year now. One thing my husband adored about his daughter was that she was a happy child.

At age three, Tobe was diagnosed with genu recurvatum (hyperextension of the knee). This was another tough period for us. However, there was a need to seek a third opinion. This time around, I discovered a doctor outside our state of residence. There was only one option left: to travel outside the state and seek another medical expert.

At this point, we were tired. We didn't want to continue with another surgery. Tobe was never able to walk independently. She had never walked barefoot as well, and it was necessary that another doctor attend to her. My husband and I later agreed to go for it. It was my husband who took our daughter for the treatment in another state. It took four months to complete the treatment. My husband would travel home after each casting. The journey was an eight-hour journey by road.

The day Tobe was supposed to go in for the Achilles tenotomy, she was not happy. She was not given a general anesthesia to keep her asleep during the procedure. Tobe was awake all through the surgery; she wailed and wailed. The nurses could not hold her, so they called for her father. My husband had to move into the operation room to hold Tobe. Eventually, she became tired of wailing and fell asleep.

My husband watched as the doctor and nurses operated on his daughter. It was not a good experience for him. The doctor and nurses did everything they had to do.

After the surgery, my husband brought Tobe back home. They traveled by road. Tobe was traumatized; she cried and cried. She just wanted to be home.

My husband was there for his daughter. If not for his intervention, the tenotomy would have been stopped halfway.

During this time, I put to bed (gave birth).

Treatment in Another Country

Tobe's treatment continued. Now, she and her twin sister had a younger sibling. I was still nursing the baby.

When Tobe was four years old, there was a need to take her to the United States for another treatment. I found an expert doctor online, Dr. D.! He invited Tobe over for treatment, and since I was still nursing my child, my husband had to go with her. They prepared for the journey and took off.

For the treatment, Tobe and her father stayed in the United States for two months, and Tobe's father played a significant role all the while.

Tobe did not like the food served on the plane; she preferred liquid, so she took only juice during the 18-hour flight. The smell of the plane food nauseated her. Every time she smelled it, she felt like throwing up. My husband had to help keep her from throwing up on the plane.

After they alighted from the plane, Tobe still felt nauseous. She rejected all the food served her in the hotel for the two months they stayed. My husband had to look for alternatives. Finally, he found some Nigerian food vendors. This was where he bought food for Tobe to eat, or he prepared the meals himself.

During the treatment, my husband did all the hospital visitations alone, beginning with the cast removal all the way through to the tenotomy days. He took Tobe to the hospital to see the doctor. He made sure Tobe ate well and had fun too. He also took her to some nice tourist spots, like visiting the zoo. Tobe had a great experience.

The US treatment worked and Tobe was healed. Now, Tobe can run, jump, and play on her own without any assistance.

My husband really played a great role in the healing story of his daughter. He truly is the Super Dad who saved the day.

approaching the end
of bnb

Maureen Hoff

WE ARE APPROACHING the end of the road. Our cutie will turn five in a few months and will graduate from her boots and bar (BnB) nightly wear. I think I am supposed to feel excited or accomplished, or even thrilled, but in reality, my feelings are more complex than that.

From the moment the first cast was placed on her foot, my cutie and I have been on a journey together. She couldn't do it without me and I wouldn't be doing this without her. We both had a clear role to play, her as the patient and me as the caregiver. We have both settled into these roles accordingly. We have established routines, clear boundaries, and expected outcomes, and we have both played our parts.

She has been a more resilient, strong, and understanding patient than I could have hoped for. Before she was born, my mind swirled with visions of fighting to keep her BnB on. Of sleeping on her floor night after night to ensure she didn't try to remove them on her own. I envisioned constant arguments and negotiations to get her to wear her BnB. Maybe even bribery; anything to make sure she met the bracing protocol.

None of those visions came to pass. The BnB became her nightly routine: no fighting, no screaming, no trying to remove the boots herself; just complete compliance with the only thing she had ever known. Even after feverish nights where we left them off to keep her temperature down, she didn't fight it when the BnB reappeared the next night. She made it look easy.

My journey as her caregiver was fraught with self-doubt, constant questioning, sleepless nights, fears of relapse, and certainties that I was doing absolutely nothing right. While my visions of a daughter fighting her treatment danced in my head, I had no visions of what I would become as her mom. I couldn't picture a mom who would advocate, question, fight for, and persevere through her daughter's yearslong treatment. I had no idea who I would become.

Just as my daughter had surprised me with her ability to cope with her BnB every night, I surprised myself with my complete capability to be her mom. I don't mean that I did everything right, that I was a perfect mom and caregiver, because I didn't, and I wasn't. But when all else failed, I was her mom.

I always seemed to find a way to figure it out for the both of us. We were a team. I was leader, and I took the role seriously. If there was a question that needed to be answered, I didn't relent until I had the answer I needed. We found our way together.

Now we find ourselves at the end of the treatment road. Our cutie is thrilled that she will be able to sleep "with just her feet," just as her older sisters do. It is sure to be one hell of a celebration; we're having big talks about what we will do. The light at the end of the tunnel draws closer and closer by each passing day, and it feels different than I thought it would.

I am thrilled for her to be through this part of treatment, but it is also bittersweet in a sense because it marks the end of a journey we have been on together. Maybe it is like when you send your child off to kindergarten for the first time. You are excited for them to grow, learn, and change, but you are sad that they will never return to a place where they were not in school. Our cutie will never return to BnB. While she may need to have different treatment ahead, it won't be years of BnB again.

The end of the road marks a change in our roles. I won't be a caregiver anymore; I will just be her mom. We have been on a long journey together and our experiences have been intertwined in a way I could never imagine. We each played our part. She was a resilient and strong patient, while I was a consistent and diligent caregiver.

When she graduates from BnB, we will find new roles to fill. Maybe she will be the soccer player and I will be her cheerleader. Or she will be the star of the show and I will be her spectator. One thing I know for certain is that she will face challenges and I will be there to support her no matter what.

Her clubfoot treatment journey created a special bond that cannot be broken and will carry us through the remainder of her life. While her BnB wear has come to an end, the lessons we have learned from her treatment will carry on forever. Because as the world constantly changes, I am forever her mom.

the humans we were meant to be

Ann-Jeanette England

OUR CLUBFOOT STORY is simply ours. It isn't the best. It isn't the worst. It is just ours. Like all, it is one worth telling. There are moments of triumph, moments of struggles, moments of unbelievable joy, and moments of unbearable heartbreak. Our journey has molded our lives. We see the world through a lens we never expected. The struggles and the victories are developing us to be the people we were meant to be. The journey is continuously evolving and shaping us to be the humans this world *needs* us to be. Through this journey our ears have heard unrecognized messages, our minds have marveled at unexpected gifts, and our hearts have been graced by unforgettable hope.

Unrecognized Messages

Our story begins with Aaron's birth. I know that sounds funny, because so many clubfoot stories start months before birth. Ours starts here. Despite numerous ultrasounds, my son's clubfoot was not discovered until he was born. Even more accurately, the discovery came a few hours later. When this amazing human was born, the medical professionals present didn't initially make any comment and didn't offer any information regarding clubfoot.

Enraptured, I stared at his face in amazement for several hours. When I finally started asking questions, I didn't get answers. I got nurses whispering amongst themselves in the corner. (By the way, I am a nurse. I know whispers are bad news. I also learned never, ever, to do this to a patient!)

I was promised someone else would answer my questions about these two tiny feet that quite obviously were not in typical position. That promised person did not come until the next day. When I finally did get information, it was provided by an aloof pediatrician who kept repeating, "It's going to be okay, everything is going to be okay." I remember very clearly that Aaron's bilateral clubfoot was so severe that, when the hospital staff attempted to change a diaper, they struggled to keep poop off his feet. I watched with skepticism as these seasoned newborn nurses struggled and thought to myself, "How are you telling me this is going to be okay while you can't even change his diaper?"

I have enough faith to know that, in general, things are going to be okay. What I needed to hear in that moment was *how. How was it was going to be okay? What was life going to look like? What was the treatment going to be? What should I expect? What does "okay" mean to you, Mr. Doctor Man?!*

Throughout our journey, the same well-intended encouragements have often left me empty. My processing and coping mechanisms simply do not work like that. Telling me that it is going to be okay, when it doesn't feel okay, does not make *me* feel okay.

To face this challenge, I developed a skill. I trained myself to start hearing the unrecognized message. When I was told, "It is going to be okay," I allowed myself to hear: "Your *feelings* are okay." "Your *fear* is okay." "*You* are okay." "You are more than okay, you are a *great* parent, even if you are *scared* or *worried* or *frustrated*." "Being sad is okay." "Celebrating the little wins is okay." "It is okay to *not want to hear* that it will be okay."

The unrecognized message that every parent needs to hear, not just clubfoot parents, is this: even when it is hard, you are a great parent because you love your child and that is what your child needs more than anything else. Your fear, doubt, worry, frustration, or sorrow do not rob you of your love for your child. Those moments of real feelings do not detract from your joy, your love, or your gratefulness for your child. Your love is what your child needs. Your love is *how* it is all going to be okay.

Unexpected Gifts

The topic of challenges typically surfaces quickly when discussing our clubfoot journey. After a complicated treatment with initial casting, difficulty with the initial tenotomy when Aaron was an infant, boots and bar bracing *long* after the typical time frame, we found that he needed additional treatment. Most people refer to it as "relapse." I prefer the term "residual deformity." A residual deformity means there are problems in the foot that are still occurring because the typical treatment plan could not completely resolve them. We were not receiving the optimal standard of care by providers in our local area, so for six years we traveled over 700 miles every three months for treatment. Due to the residual deformity causing problems with Aaron's ability to walk and run properly, we sought the counsel of another highly recommended provider, also hundreds of miles from home.

The time between visits consisted of extra time in boots and bar, physical therapy and stretching. Aaron worked *hard* in physical therapy. We were stretching regularly with a very regimented schedule. With all of this stretching and bracing, it often seemed like we never slept. Despite our diligence and Aaron's hard work, there was a pit in my stomach. My gut was telling me that something wasn't right. I don't think anyone watches their kids walk with the same intensity as clubfoot parents. I dissected every step he took and that pit grew heavier. I wanted so desperately to be wrong. I wasn't.

Before I knew it, I found myself sitting in front of the doctor, faced with the confirmation of what I feared the most. I was alone with Aaron at this appointment. Someone asked me what it was like to hear that the residual deformity needed treatment. It felt like a ton of bricks. I should have been prepared. I should have known. And yet, there it was: a ton of bricks.

We started discussing the treatment options. The doctor told us that we needed to proceed with bilateral anterior tibialis tendon transfer surgeries and another Achilles tenotomy. This would mean that our treatment plan now involved traveling *2,000 miles* away from home. We would need to travel from California to St. Louis, Missouri. As we discussed the treatment plan, I felt isolated in the moment. It was as if the world had stopped in its tracks yet was spinning faster than ever around me at the same time. I could not seem to get a grip on anything.

Aaron was six years old at the time; it was the summer before he was starting first grade. In my mind, this was the worst possible time that we could interrupt his schooling. I remember thinking about how he had just started making friends in kindergarten. I had an understanding that first grade is an important foundational year. For a moment, I believed this news was tragic.

I knew that we needed to do it. I knew it was something that we would get through. I knew it was something that we would become stronger from; nevertheless, I was really sad and frustrated that *this* was what we needed to do. I was scared. Fortunately, our doctor was remarkably wonderful. She had a plan and she explained everything that we needed to know. She told us that he would need to be in a wheelchair and the length of time we would need for recovery. Not only is this provider a *brilliant* practitioner, but also her bedside manner is a skill she has developed well. In the midst of my storm of fear, she was a cool and calm breeze of peace.

My son is inquisitive and very aware of his entire clubfoot journey and treatment process. He paid close attention during the appointment. He was also very quiet, which, if you know Aaron, is a rare event! As we walked out of the appointment, I asked him how much he understood of everything that she said. He just looked at me. The world stopped spinning for a moment and he just looked at me. I sat down on the floor to be eye level with him. His eyes appeared deep and dark. He seemed so much older than six at that moment. It was like his soul was reaching out to mine.

Finally, he drew in a long breath, let it out slowly. His eyes stayed locked on mine, and he said, "Mom, I know this is what we need to do. I am ready to do it. I just *really, really* want to do it before I turn seven."

I did not know what to say. I was so proud of Aaron for accepting the responsibility of doing something that he knew was going to be difficult. I had this overwhelming pride for his ability to articulate what he was feeling and to communicate wanting to have the procedure done before he turned seven years old. This part may not seem like a big deal, but it was complicated. This timeline only gave us about seven months. Due to some recent changes in health insurance, I was not confident the seven months would be sufficient time to get the treatment approved and completed. By the grace of God, were able to proceed right away.

We made three trips to St. Louis, traveling over 12,000 miles. Aaron was amazing! He remained positive despite many challenges in traveling and in his treatment. I'm so proud of how strong he is. He never felt sorry for himself. He embraced his journey, and his compassion for others has grown tremendously along the way.

The next part of our story is particularly special because of the tight time frame in which all of this transpired. The appointment with the provider I just described took place in June 2019. Aaron proceeded with his tenotomy and tendon transfer surgery in October 2019. His last cast came off in late December 2019. Aaron turned seven in January 2020. Because of the circumstances with health insurance, had Aaron not made the request to have surgery before his birthday, we probably would have delayed the treatment until after January 2020. We could have never predicted that in February 2020 the world would change dramatically with the Covid pandemic. Had we waited and not completed the surgery before January 2020, I would be telling a very different story right now. His entire treatment program would have been significantly influenced and delayed. There could have been a tremendous impact on the outcome and prognosis.

To this day, I am astounded at the intuition that my son had and the bravery that he demonstrated in expressing his feelings after that appointment. This unexpected gift he has been given, this incredible intuition, is a source of splendor in our story. This is what I believe is so inspirational about children with clubfoot. Not only are they resilient, strong, and brave, but also, through the challenges in their clubfoot journey, so many other wondrous gifts blossom in our children. Some clubfoot kids develop an amazing sense of humor because of this journey, and that is a character trait to celebrate. Others mature into incredibly determined individuals with perseverance to accomplish anything. The gifts are there within these children waiting for the opportunity to shine bright.

When I think about this unexpected gift we discovered through this journey, I am reminded of what an amazing person my child is. At six years old, he listened to his inner self, and he communicated what he heard. This moment allowed me to see him for all the brilliance he possesses. It helped me see this journey for more than the challenges. I see the journey for the beauty it unveils along the way. This journey is part of THE journey for my son. This is what is developing him into the amazing human he is becoming every day. I get to be on this journey with him; I get the front-row seat! What this moment made me realize is that I don't want my kids to be who I imagined. They are already so much greater than anything I could have imaged or expected. What a gift!

Unforgettable Hope

It turns out, hope can be found in a giant pile of puffy pillows. If you have had a bigger kid with residual (relapse) treatment with long leg casts, you know that pillows (*lots and lots of pillows*) are required. More pillows than you ever thought could fit on a bed, and then a few more.

While we were in St. Louis for Aaron's surgeries, we were staying in a hotel. The hotel was not our original plan. However, due to some unfortunate circumstances, this is where we were. As hotels go, it was nice. It was clean, the staff was friendly, it fit our needs. As our journey would have it, this hotel provided for us in ways we never could have expected. Our hospital experience for the surgery was not smooth. Think anesthesia issues, nursing issues, overcrowded hospital issues—you name it. We struggled to keep his pain under control, and while I am sympathetic to over-worked nursing staff, we found very little compassion in the hospital. I often found myself wishing we could be discharged early so that we could return to the hotel, where I could care for my son myself.

When Aaron was finally discharged and we were back at the hotel, a new set of challenges emerged. Aaron struggled significantly with pain after the surgeries, more so than what I'm told the average child does. We responded with pain meds and pillows. We were constantly trying to fluff up his bed, elevate his legs, shove pillows anywhere and everywhere we could to try to make our son more comfortable.

Our constant need for pillows meant nearly hourly calls to the hotel staff requesting, you guessed it, more pillows. The hotel staff *never* acted too busy, too irritated, or too frustrated with us. They brought us more pillows at every request. Aaron experienced severe muscle cramps and intermittent bursts of pain. When this would happen, he would wake up screaming. I worried that his crying in pain disturbed other guests. I imagined the complaints fielded by the staff.

One day there was a knock on the door, and I feared we had worn out the patience of the staff and guests. Instead, what I found was evidence of hope for humanity. The housekeeping staff stood before me. The same housekeeping staff tasked with making trips to and from our room to bring extra pillows on a near constant rotation were standing in front of me. This time, they were not holding pillows, but a basket of goodies for my son. The housekeepers had taken up a collection and put together a basket of coloring books, crayons, candy, Gatorade, and several other items a six-year-old might enjoy. They placed all these gifts of love into a basket and wrapped it up with a bow.

The people who had the most justification for being frustrated with us and could have come with complaints about noise, brought love instead. The women standing at the door explained that they had all been watching since the first day we returned from the hospital. They said their hearts broke for how much pain he must be experiencing. One woman said she watched from an upstairs window as we struggled to get him out of the car, and she melted with compassion for him. They expressed how, with every trip to bring us pillows, instead of growing in frustration, they grew in compassion.

If you ask me, *this moment*, this moment with these humans showing compassion and love to my family in our time of need, *this moment*, will forever be one of the greatest moments in all of history. I have absolutely no doubt that this moment will forever shape how my family responds to the needs of others. I have already witnessed my son and daughter refuse to walk away from someone in need of compassion. The greatness in this act of humanity poured over my son in our darkest moments is a pinnacle moment not only in our clubfoot journey, but in our lives. This moment of unforgettable hope is a beacon in our journey. I cannot write these words without tears of gratitude filling my oh-so-tired eyes. The light of this moment of human greatness drowns the shadows of all the moments of doubt, fear, and worry.

Perhaps the most remarkable thing about our story is beauty within the struggle. Don't get me wrong—I don't always think it is beautiful, but it is. It is hard, but it is also miraculous. Just like all the other stories of incredible children and dedicated parents, the beauty is found in what we never imagined our story would be. When I was pregnant and imagining what life with this little human was going to be like, I did not comprehend the depth this life would have for us. This journey allows us to open ourselves up to be the humans we were meant to be. I get to watch my child triumph over incredible challenges.

We have discovered that we were made for so much more than just surviving the difficult times. We were created to thrive in the midst of storms. We have met the most remarkable people who have brought unforgettable hope into our lives. We are regularly encouraged by unrecognized messages. Unexpected gifts have been revealed to us as our child blossoms. It is very easy to picture a diagnosis like clubfoot as a fence that will limit your life experiences. What we have discovered is that what looks like a fence is truly a gate that opens to a world of unbelievable possibilities.

You can find Ann-Jeannette's son Aaron's story, "Clubfoot: The Incredible Journey," in the next section on page 93.

if i had a crystal ball

Allie Zimmerman

IT'S BEEN NEARLY 14 years since we heard the words "there are some birth defects that have us concerned." I remember the perinatologist coming in, pulling up the ultrasound and looking at my baby's brain, her heart, back to her brain, down to her legs and feet, back to her brain, to her feet. Asking me several times who my OB/GYN was. I had heard *of* clubfeet but never really heard *about* clubfeet. He told us she'd barely be able to walk, that she'd do PE but likely never be able to keep up with her peers.

After an amniocentesis to rule out any other conditions, we were told the baby had clubfeet and curved pinkies, no other underlying conditions. We were given a list of names to interview prior to her arrival. One doctor was old and impatient and never took his hand off the door his entire consult with us, one gave us the heebie-jeebies, and then there was the one my daughter would later refer to as Dr. Fluffy Unicorn, a name he earned after her first surgery and several doses of morphine. He was the one I knew would give her the best life possible. He was the one I trusted with her future.

Riley arrived, all 4 lbs and 14 oz of her, four weeks early with a set of lungs that cleared the room and two perfectly imperfect feet. Ten days later, we showed up to Dr. Fluffy Unicorn's office and the magic began. She was still likely under 5 lbs, but he manipulated her feet, and she barely ever made a peep. His office administrator would scoop her up each visit and walk her around the office so I could catch my breath. She was an equally huge part of Riley's treatment as Dr. Fluffy Unicorn was. She made that office our family—something I would later look back on and realize how important that was in Riley's treatment. It was a safe place, a place where I knew they would take care of our girl like she was their own. We sailed through casting, brace, and bar with zero issues, so at three years old, she graduated from brace wear.

We had a few years of great checkups. Then one day, she was walking in flip-flops and I just knew the relapse that we dreaded so much had arrived. Shoes disguised her regression, but flip-flops showed it all: a heel that never touched the ground, the foot turning in with each step. She had bruises on her legs from falling when she was running because her gait was off due to the regression.

We got her in to see the doctor a few weeks later. Sure enough, he confirmed the regression in her left foot. We started serial casting to correct her foot. She made progress, but a few weeks after each cast we saw her foot regress again. At age five, Riley had a tendon transfer on her left foot.

The total feeling of failing as a mom hit me like a ton of bricks. Everything had gone so smoothly through treatment. What if I had kept her in her braces longer? What if I was more diligent with her stretches? Dr. Fluffy Unicorn had tears in his eyes as he gave us the recommendation for surgery. He offered to send us for a second opinion, but I knew in my heart that the anterior tibialis tendon transfer (ATTT) surgery was what she needed. The frequent casts took a toll on her mental health, took her out of the sports she loved and craved. At age eight, her right foot regressed and she had the tendon transfer on that foot. That one I took a little better since I knew the amazing outcome she'd had on her left foot, but sending your kid into major surgery is never easy on the heart.

When Riley was about 10, Dr. Fluffy Unicorn stopped practicing. She was heartbroken, as was I. Dr Fluffy Unicorn, well, he was a unicorn. He taught her to advocate for herself and her feet, he let her be a kid first and scheduled surgeries around her sports schedule. He cried when he told us she needed her first surgery, and later, he was the one who came up with guided growth surgery because it would only take her out of softball for a few weeks and was minimally invasive. My momma heart couldn't put her through an invasive surgery after living through a pandemic and finally getting back to school and sports. Riley and Dr. Fluffy Unicorn still text each other here and there. And he will forever be the doctor that Riley and I compare all other doctors to. She's been known to leave an orthopedic office and say, "He's okay but he's no Dr. Fluffy Unicorn."

At this point, it was clear that Riley's feet were stubborn. Finally, at age 12 she had guided growth surgery on both feet to try to make her Achilles lengthen without an invasive surgery. We hope this is her last surgery. She's been to PT, she's worn nighttime braces in some form until she was 13—it's been a journey. A long, grueling journey.

Despite the long journey she's been on, Riley is now in eighth grade. She's your typical teen. She loves shoes, friends, and softball; her parents are mortifying; she really loves softball; she's in National Junior Honor Society; and did I mention she loves softball? She sleeps, eats, breathes, and dreams softball. She plays competitive travel softball with dreams of playing in college and even in the Olympics (and Dr. Fluffy Unicorn dreams of making the cover of *Sports Illustrated* with her). She does F45 fitness training when I drag her with me. She does speed and agility; her squats are questionable at best due to her tight Achilles tendon, but every day she's 1% better. Yet she only has a handful of pictures of where her feet started. I was so focused on getting her "fixed" that I didn't think about the marvel of her transformation.

If I had a crystal ball, I'd tell my past self to take all the pictures of her natural feet. That one day she'd turn into a confident young lady who has exceeded expectations and she'll want to show friends, teammates, coaches, and teachers where she began. She's the kid that wears her scars as badges of honor, naming off where each surgery left its mark, even the now tiny barely visible scars from her tenotomy at three months old.

I'd tell my past self that some days it won't be okay. Some days you'll wonder, *why us? Why her? When is this going to be over?* Some days you'll have a pity party and cry yourself to sleep because clubfeet were supposed to be over at age five and it's still going strong at 13, and you'll worry incessantly about her future. Some days it's just not okay. And that's okay. You have a baby with a birth defect: it's okay to not be okay. But one day that feisty little girl who was born with two crooked feet will turn to you and say, "But Mom, I can't help that I was made to run." One day she'll come home and tell you that she beat the boys who were being mean to her in a race. You'll see her step onto the softball field and hit an inside-the-park home run. Or you'll see her steal base after base, or hear a coach comment on her speed. Or she'll pop from her catcher's squat and toss a runner out who was trying to steal on her. And all of those things will make your heart burst with happiness because you know where she started and you think, "It will all be okay," and slowly those hard days fade away and become a distant memory.

And by the way ... she hit her inside-the-park home run, she steals base after base, and no runner dares steal on her because her pop-up is faster than the best of the best.

You can find Allie's daughter Riley's story, "Big Goals," in the next section on page 98.

grief and dreams

Lori T. Howard

NOTHING PREPARES you for the day a doctor comes in to tell you that something will be wrong with the baby you are carrying. Before that day, I had imagined a perfect baby who would do great and amazing things and whose life would be easy and free from pain. That is, after all, what we all want for our children.

At my 20-week ultrasound, I was told not only would my baby have bilateral clubfeet, but also that she had a giant hole in her heart and most likely had trisomy 13—a chromosomal condition that makes it impossible to survive outside the womb.

When I heard those words, my dream of the life my baby would have came crashing down. I was thrust into a world of science and doctors and all sorts of procedures I had not only never heard of, but also never dreamed that I, a very healthy young mother, would ever have to endure.

As soon as baby Chloe was born, and the doctors determined that her heart and chromosomes were all okay, my husband and I breathed a collective sigh of relief. We were only dealing with one clubfoot and that was fixable, right? We live in the age of modern medicine and scientific studies. I had heard that Olympic soccer player Mia Hamm and Olympic ice skater Kristi Yamaguchi had clubfeet. So, really, how bad could it be?

But, for Chloe, living with a unilateral clubfoot has been not only a physically painful journey, but an emotionally scarring one as well.

As her mother, watching her navigate the doctor's visits, surgeries, and bullying because of her disability became the greatest challenge of my life.

You see, the truth of having a child with a disability is that it is often the mother who carries the weight of the emotional impact, as well as the caregiving for the child. There is nothing a mother would not do for her baby, and for a child with a disability, a mother, and I mean ME here, would do anything.

When Chloe was born, something clicked inside me that turned on my inner lioness—that feeling that no one was ever going to hurt my child without going through me first. While I know this is a common thing that happens after the birth of a baby, for a mother of a child with a disability, it is further impacted because we know how cruel the world is to even typical kids. We want to do everything in our power to make sure our kid has a pain-free life. We are here to shape our children, to protect them while they grow up, and much like the boots and bar that Chloe had to wear, our job, as mothers, is to gently guide our children into adulthood with as little scarring as possible.

Chloe started having casting on her clubfoot at two weeks old. Her doctor in San Francisco was determined to manipulate her foot using castings. By the time Chloe was six months old, it was obvious that her foot was not responsive to the treatment. The doctor decided that surgery to transfer her tendon was the way to go. Unfortunately, this doctor was not trained in the Ponseti method. After Chloe's surgery at six months, not only was the mobility of her foot now frozen in place due to the tendon transfer, but it started to regress and turn inward again.

What that looked like for a new young mother was holding crying Chloe down for weekly cast changes. Nursing infant Chloe who had a diaper-to-toe plaster cast on. Watching six-month-old

Chloe waking up from surgery crying out from the pain, which was only subdued by her morphine drip. It was hard. It was scary. And it made me a very anxious mom.

We were lucky enough to move to Seattle when Chloe was one, where we found a new orthopedist. This doctor was considered the clubfoot guru of the West and was trained in Ponseti. He quickly began casting Chloe again. Chloe learned to walk, much later than the typical child, dragging a huge cast around. Then we started using the boots and bar that she would also drag around while her foot was learning a new way to grow. We were hopeful that it would make a difference. And Chloe, being that she was the most easygoing baby, was amenable to all of this.

She fell asleep with her "night-night shoes" on every night. When my husband and I took a very rare date night out, I had to prep the babysitter on how to make sure the shoes were on correctly.

Chloe never complained. She rarely cried out in distress when her feet were squeezed into the shoes. She often laughed during cast changes because Elmo was always on the screen. I told her that she was perfect in her imperfection and that she was beautifully made. We always filled her up with positive reinforcement so she could see the world as a safe and beautiful place. Like the boots and bar reshaping her feet, I was trying to cement in her mind that she was perfect just the way she was.

I, on the other hand, was filled with anxiety that Chloe would not be able to participate in activities like her peers or be accepted by them.

At age three, her doctor realized that the Ponseti method wasn't working as expected due to her prior surgery, and she needed another major surgery. This time, the doctor repositioned her foot and she went through more rounds of casting and boots and bars after that.

By age five, Chloe's foot still wouldn't stay straight. She wore her casts proudly to kindergarten. She had many rounds of casting and boots and bars. Chloe would get her cast off, have swim lessons, get the cast back on, and see how it went. She managed swim lessons, learning to ride a bike, and pony riding through it all.

When you have a child with a disability, the everyday stuff is more difficult. I could never forget the boots and bar for fear her foot would regress. I became very regimented in sleep patterns and naptime—because those were hours where her foot could heal. I learned the ins and outs of hospitals and doctors' offices and had to learn how to navigate her wheelchair after surgeries.

When Chloe was seven years old, we moved back to California and found an orthopedist at the University of California San Francisco (UCSF) hospital who happened to be the student of our guru doctor. It became clear, again, that more surgery was needed. So, in fourth grade, Chloe had an osteotomy and bone fusion. This is one of the most painful surgeries one can have—when the doctor cuts through bone to repair something and then adds donor bone to help. After this surgery, Chloe had a harder recovery. This meant that I was her nurse, once again, and my life revolved around doctor visits and wound care.

Fast forward to seventh grade. Chloe's legs were now different lengths. To help with the leg-length discrepancy, the doctor decided to stunt the growth in her good leg so her clubfoot leg could catch up. That meant she needed a surgical procedure on the growth plate of her good leg, called an epiphysiodesis. Once again, I was ready with the wheelchair, the wound tending, and the constant hovering.

I kept worrying about Chloe. Was she happy? Was she making friends? Did people accept her? In the back of my mind, I felt like I had to make sure that Chloe was accepted—even though that is not something any mom can do. My worst fears were realized when she was assaulted at age 14 by a group of peers because of her difference. It was as if I was also assaulted. It felt like all of my care and work to help Chloe feel like a typical kid was lost at that moment. Her grief became mine. It was a hard time.

That same year, Chloe had to have screws and metal plates taken out of her leg due to the pain they were causing. Her leg hadn't grown the length we wanted it to, which felt like another blow. Yet, Chloe soldiered on. She was determined to fight through it. I, on the other hand, was getting weary.

As Chloe finished her high school years, I finally found space to spend some time focusing on myself. I went back to school and am now a licensed psychotherapist, which helped with my own issues. Now, I work with families who have children with special needs, as well as many other areas of grief and loss. Because what I have come to realize is that when you have a child with a disability, it is a loss for a parent. Parents have expectations of what our children will be, and having a clubfoot is not in that expectation.

When Chloe went away to college, it was another blow for me. My life's work as Chloe's mom/nurse was ending and it took me a few months to navigate the new loss. But, as before, Chloe's foot had other ideas. Another unexpected surgery happened when Chloe's deformed toe bone decided to bore through her skin. So, I was back to helping my 18-year-old daughter bathe, get dressed, and navigate her world. But this time, we shared a lot of laughter and joy in the process. I was no longer afraid that the world would not accept Chloe—she had grown into a strong and resilient woman of her own. I was able to care for her not out of a need to protect, but because I was just being a typical mom—and it felt good.

Twenty-two years after Chloe's traumatic entrance to the world, I can tell you that my initial dream of having a child who was physically perfect and who would experience no pain in life did not come true. Instead, Chloe has grown into a young woman who is far beyond any dream or hope I could have imagined. And I know it is partly because of my care of her emotional and physical well-being.

We cannot protect our children from pain. We cannot protect our children from physical deformity or mental illness, or bullies or pretty much most things. But we can show up for them and be their cheering squad when life is difficult.

Having a child with a clubfoot is hard. It isn't what any mother dreams about when they envision what their future children will be like. But it is also not the end of a dream. Ultimately, my dream for Chloe was that she would grow up to be a strong woman who knows who she is, is kind, and loves others. Her foot is one small part of her story, and mine. Our stories are still being written, and it is a joy and honor to share my story with my daughter.

You can find Lori's daughter Chloe's story, "Just Chloe," in the next section on page 100.

walking through life with clubfoot

We are happy to be able to include some perspectives in this book about the experience of growing up while dealing with residual clubfoot. Residual clubfoot requires additional treatment beyond the typical Ponseti method. The Ponseti method minimizes surgery, but in the past, surgery was more common. In two of these perspectives, you'll hear from adults who were children in the 1960s and '70s, and the surgical treatments they underwent.

For those readers who have babies with clubfoot, your child will likely have an easier time than this. When treatment goes smoothly, many people who were born with clubfoot don't think about it much when they're older kids or adults. For instance, when Betsy asked a friend if he wanted to write about his clubfoot experience for this book, he responded that he didn't remember much about it. He just knew he was treated in early childhood. He said clubfoot hadn't affected his life much, so he didn't have a story to tell.

clubfoot: the incredible journey

Aaron England

MY NAME IS Aaron and I am nine years old. I am going to tell you about the biggest adventures of my life—let's get started. One of my first memories regarding clubfoot treatment is one of my favorites. For many years we have traveled hundreds of miles for visits with my doctors. On several of these trips Papa (my grandpa) came with us to keep my mom and me company.

Mom made a tradition, and nearly every trip, we visited the beach, even if just for a few minutes. One time when I was three years old, Papa and I wanted to put our feet in the water. We kept saying we would only get in *"to our ankles."* We didn't have towels or extra clothes with us. Before we knew it, Papa and I were both soaked. Mom likes to tease us that we always cause trouble because of this day. We all still laugh about it. It is one of my favorite memories ever, not just in my clubfoot journey.

When I was six years old, I started hearing my doctor talk about "relapse." The doctor and my mom discussed something like a procedure. I knew I probably had to go through surgery. Mom and I went outside after the appointment and sat on the floor.

Mom said, "Buddy, did you just hear that you are going to have to have a surgery on your feet?"

I was more shocked than ever before in my life—but I had this feeling that I was going to get through it. Before the surgery, I would need multiple casts. After the surgery, I had long leg casts again and then short casts. Despite the journey ahead of me, I was proud of myself for accepting the challenges.

We traveled several hours many times to visit the doctor for cast changes and checkups. We flew from California to St. Louis, Missouri, three times. I wasn't scared. I was really excited to travel. I had the awesome opportunity to meet many different people. Almost everyone encouraged me. People would talk to me about my casts and wheelchair. I got to teach a lot people about club-foot. I also learned a lot from the people I met. I often think that if I didn't have these surgeries, I would have missed a lot of great adventures.

St. Louis is near the Mississippi River with many amazing people and places to visit. I absolutely loved visiting a famous landmark called the Gateway Arch. An elevator takes you up about 600 feet. It is an amazing experience to look out from such a high point. I would encourage anyone thinking about visiting the Arch to make it a priority. It is a remarkable place and not scary at all.

At the St. Louis Science Center, we went to the planetarium. I felt like I was actually under the stars. I love science, so the visits to the Science Center are incredible memories for me. The time I spent there fed my love of science. I learned so much.

The St. Louis Zoo holds many wonderful memories for my family and me. We would visit the animals often. It helped distract me from the discomfort of the treatment with casts and the surgery. There were polar bears, grizzly bears, red pandas, and so many more unique animals. I loved seeing the animals. As I watched them, my worries and fears seemed to drift away.

St. Louis is home to a place called the City Museum. This memory stands out because it is an adventure unlike any other I have ever had. It is a difficult place to describe. Small pathways, ladders, and tubes lead all over a building. You can crawl in and out of these passageways going up and down several floors through creative and interesting maze-type obstacles. There is even a 10-story slide. Adventures were around every corner, literally.

The flights were an adventure themselves. People were remarkably kind and showed me so much compassion. Many people wanted to talk to me because of the casts. Several told me that they had a friend or family member with clubfoot. It was really fun talking to people. I was able to spend a lot of time with the flight crew. I asked a lot of questions about the airplane engines, the fuel, and flight plans. With each flight I learned more and more. I will always remember talking with so many people, learning so much, and feeling the compassion of everyone around me.

At home, while I was recovering from surgery and in the wheelchair, a friend of my mom made special arrangements for me. She had friends at the California Highway Patrol who allowed me to visit the station where they kept the helicopter. I asked *so* many questions. I got to see the inside and outside of the helicopter up close. I watched it take off and land. A few days later, they flew the helicopter over my house and talked to me over the loudspeaker. It caused quite a scare with some of the neighbors. It was an unbelievable experience that I will never forget.

When I went through my surgeries, I was in first grade. You might think that kids at school would bully me because of the wheelchair and casts, but that did not happen. It was the opposite, actually. Everyone was nice to me. I could not have asked for a better experience at school. Kids in my class brought me a stuffed bear in a wheelchair.

Having to be in a wheelchair wasn't all bad. It was quite fun to zoom around twice as fast as I would normally run. It was also super fun to give my sister rides on the back of the wheelchair. Behind the seat of the wheelchair, there are foot pegs used to keep the chair from tipping backward. My sister would stand on these pegs and get rides from me nearly everywhere we went. I always told her that the step tracker on her watch was reduced by probably 5,000 steps every day.

My teacher was incredible. She let me teach my class about clubfoot. She took my desk apart and adjusted the height to help me be more comfortable. I found encouraging notes from her in my homework that she prepared for my long trips for treatment. The school arranged for upper-grade students to earn community service credits for pushing my wheelchair at school. It was nice to have a break from pushing myself, but it was even better to have someone to talk to and pass the time with. I couldn't go play at recess, so the upper-grade students talked with me and played board games. I experienced great kindness at my school, which will live in my heart forever.

I am telling the stories of all these wonderful adventures to encourage kids and parents. You might be thinking to yourself *the clubfoot journey is very difficult.* I want to show the positive side of the journey. The treatment was hard, being in casts was hard, but it was also a great adventure.

I often think about kids around the world who don't have the option of treatment. Sometimes families don't have enough money, or treatment isn't available near them. This is why I like to support other kids. I do fundraisers every year to help kids receive clubfoot treatment. I want all children to have a good life. I want them to experience the good things I have experienced. Helping others also helps me remember in the hard times that I am fortunate to receive treatment. I am fortunate to have adventures because of the treatment. I had a lot of pain after the surgeries, but I am grateful for the treatment. I am grateful for the opportunities my clubfoot journey has given me and will give me in life.

I want to encourage parents and kids. If your child is experiencing pain and difficult times, you will get through it, and it will be worth it. Clubfoot and treatment are not all about pain and struggle. Yes, there are hard times, but there are also a lot of adventures. My clubfoot journey has led me on many different adventures that I am grateful for. Those adventures are what I remember more than the struggles.

You can find Aaron's mom Ann-Jeannette's story, "The Humans We Were Meant to Be," in the previous section on page 72.

big goals

Riley Zimmerman

WHEN I WAS YOUNGER, I thought everyone went to the orthopedic surgeon. It wasn't until I was three and a half years old that my parents told me about my feet and showed me a picture of what they looked like before my doctor began correcting them. My parents explained it to me like everyone is different; some people have blond hair, some wear glasses, and some, like me, have crooked feet. Because of the way they explained it, I never let my feet get in the way of my big dreams.

Now I'm 13. Sometimes I do get scared. The fact that I have 12 incisions between both feet combined is scary. Sometimes I worry that I'll pop out my tendon transfer from my ATTT surgery. But my biggest fear is at some point in time my feet will keep me from pursuing my dreams. And I have big dreams. I want to play college softball and even play for the US Olympic team.

These worries sometimes drag me down, but I have also gained a lot from experiencing clubfoot. The doctor who diagnosed my feet before I was born told my parents that I wouldn't be able to keep up with my peers, but I excel at my sport, softball. Clubfoot has made me more sympathetic than most kids my age toward people who may be going through hard times in their lives. It has taught me that you never know what mountain people have had to climb to get to where they are. I've had to climb some pretty big mountains to compete at the level I compete at.

Sometimes I am self-conscious about my scars, but when people ask, I tell them I had surgery. It's annoying having to explain what clubfoot is. I wish people knew more about it. My goal for my journey is to educate people about clubfoot, to teach them that, with hard work, anything is possible no matter what you have to overcome. Clubfoot is my superpower; it is what makes me strong.

You can find Riley's mom Allie's story, "If I Had a Crystal Ball," in the previous section on page 81.

just chloe

Chloe Howard

MY NAME'S CHLOE, I'm 22 years old, and I was born with a
severe unilateral clubfoot. Growing up I knew that I was different: there were significant aspects of my life that set me apart from
my peers. Maybe it was that my Daddy-Daughter Dates were to
get my hot pink casts cut off, or perhaps it was that I knew what a
9/10 on the numbered pain scale felt like (I was saving my 10).
Maybe it was that I knew how to do awesome tricks in a wheelchair, and maybe it was that I was the only kid I knew at school
who was strapped into foot abduction braces (my "night-night
shoes") right before bedtime. It could have even been that I was
the only kid pulled out of the pool during swim team practice so
the coach could watch as I attempted to flutter kick effectively
with my unpointable left foot. From a very young age, I knew that
there was a very specific way my body looked and moved that was
altogether different from how everyone else's did, and that was a
rather large reality to hold.

I've had nine major surgeries to correct my clubfoot, the first
when I was six months old and the most recent when I was 18
years old. This impressive and expansive list of procedures
includes tendon transfers and bone graphs, with my osteotomy

and fusion surgery at nine years old topping the list as the most complicated and painful procedure and recovery, but the most effective in making my beautiful little foot the straightest it had ever been. These surgeries involved wheelchairs and education on many big medical words to describe what would happen to me. So, starting in elementary school, I decided that, if I was going to prepare myself for months in a wheelchair and how to describe exactly what an osteotomy was, I would prepare my peers, too. In fourth grade, I gave my first classroom presentation before that osteotomy surgery. I stood up in front of my class of 24 nine-year-olds and showed them a slideshow presentation of pictures of my feet and definitions of related words, told them what to expect when I returned to school, and how, after all this, I was still just Chloe.

This became something that empowered me: telling others about my foot, on my terms. It was important to me that people saw me as just Chloe, and that when they learned about my club-foot, in their mind it was just a cool addition to who that Chloe was. In our society, we talk a lot about the word "normal"—what it means, what it looks like, how we can achieve that standard. But we're not created to exist within parameters, and for some reason, that incredible and freeing truth wasn't something I ever really needed to be taught. I always just kind of knew I wasn't meant to fit any defined "normal." It was obvious to me that my foot was different in a way that shaped me into a specific and unique version of me that wouldn't exist in the same way if my foot wasn't the glorious messy beautiful thing that it was. And that was incredibly cool to me—that my foot was part of my story and was actively shaping the Chloe I was growing up to be.

But carrying this foot and its story with me every day isn't the easiest thing. I have pain that starts at the inner curve of my foot that wraps around my ankle and heel when I stand or walk for longer than 30 minutes. There are times at the beach when I want to hide my foot in the sand around people I don't know well. I can't wear heels taller than an inch and a half, a fact that I believed absolutely ostracized me at middle school graduation. I became a victim of hate crime assault because of my clubfoot at age 14, and despite the perpetrator's sentencing, it took me many years in therapy to reestablish the idea of my foot as safe in my mind.

I grew up in a family grounded in faith, and that faith guided me in love, patience, grace, and grit. Love for myself and the foot that was crafted and molded just for me; patience while I learned the intricacies of my foot and the beauty of my twisting scars. There was grace during the days I felt angry with my foot for not doing what I wanted it to be able to do, and there was grit to convince my occasionally scared and stubborn mind to love, and love, and love. This love, patience, grace, and grit have shaped the narrative I tell myself about my foot: there is purpose behind my pain, my foot is a part of me, not a mistake, and it is my responsibility and gift to tell a story centered around courage, confidence, and hope. Because that's what this story is.

When I was in middle school, I spent a lot of time worrying about whether the baby I might one day carry would look like me. I'd lay in my bed at night in cloud-printed pajamas and wonder if my clubfoot meant she'd have one too. Would she have blonde hair and blue eyes and a painfully twisted foot? Would she be shy and sprout little freckles in the summer and have no toenails like me? I used to wish I could allow myself to fall in love with the idea of the child I might have. Strong and beautiful and brave, eyes full of energy, and a mind that could not fathom the beauty of the world around them. But I would stop myself, my fears protecting my heart from the possibility of its breaking.

I do not know how to reconcile my hopes with my fears, my "typical" with my "abnormal," my "could be" with my "should have been." And I may never understand the complexity of the human mind and why certain patterns of thought seem to play in echoes over yearlong expanses of our lives; why 10-year-old Chloe would lay under her polka-dot duvet and wish her pain could be only hers to carry. But I do know now, aged 22 and no longer 10, that it is not my job to fear what is so far out of my control. I no longer worry about whether any future children I might have will be born with clubfeet; I will figure it out and learn as I go, as so many other incredible and courageous women have before me. I no longer worry if a guy will break up with me when he learns about my feet; I'm loved by the kindest man who rubs my foot when it hurts and even when it doesn't. I don't know why it was my foot that was twisted, why my family would carry this story alongside me—but I have found so much peace in learning that the "why" doesn't matter. It is our job to respond: for parents to love those special feet and to nurture little hearts to love them on their own, and for those with clubfeet to not allow fears, anxieties, guilt, and shame to take power over awe, wonder, curiosity, and hope.

I've learned that our stories are powerful and are ours to tell. Mothers: thousands of women around the world have children whose feet look like your child's. This reality means two things. You are not alone in your pain, your hurt, your frustration, your loneliness, your confusion, your exhaustion; and your story— your sharing of that frustration, loneliness, exhaustion—matters. And to those with clubfeet: your foot is so special. Nothing about you is an accident. You are incredibly loved, and there are so many people on your team. Believe the truth that you are beautiful and one of a kind. Life is bigger than just this moment, and it will not always be this hard, I promise.

Parents, you did nothing wrong, and you are doing the right thing. Your job at this time is to believe in your children and carry their clubfoot story with them, and I believe you are fully equipped to do so because I believe in extraordinary love and extraordinary strength. It might be scary right now, and I don't know what the future holds, but in you exists the power to believe the world is beautiful and you were created to love these special feet. So, love, and love, and love.

You can find Chloe's mom Lori's story, "Grief and Dreams," in the previous section on page 85.

why no baby pictures?

Laura (Rayl) Bucknam

THERE ARE VERY few pictures of me as a baby. There are none of my clubfeet. That may not seem odd for a child born in 1960, except that my father was a photographer. He was an Army photographer stationed at Kagnew Station, Asmara, Eritrea, Ethiopia. (Eritrea was not its own country at that time.)

When I was born, my parents were devastated to learn that I had what the doctor called "a rather severe clubfoot deformity bilaterally." The Army sent us back to the United States for evaluation and treatment. When I was two months old, both of my feet were placed in plaster casts that went the full length of my legs. My feet were treated with progressive casting until I was 17 months old. I know that they added a lot of extra weight. My mom had to care for three young girls, one of whom wore the heavy casts. After 15 months of casting, it was believed that my feet were corrected. One consequence is that I learned to walk with casts on.

We had returned to Africa when I was a year old. We were still there when, at the age of four, I was seen by the doctors again. Once again, they put casts on my legs. This time, after no significant progress in nine weeks, it was decided that we would return to the United States so that I could undergo surgery at Walter

Reed Army Medical Center in Washington, DC. That event led
to my sisters and me being raised in Manassas, Virginia.

My first surgery was done in August 1964. As a four-year-old
child, I still remember them placing a mask over my face. The
medical record states that surgery was done "under gas, oxygen,
ether, nitrous oxide, and fluothane anesthesia." It was very scary
for me to be put to sleep that way. My second surgery was four
weeks later in September. The doctors would only operate on one
foot at a time. My records indicate that the surgery involved
"release of the left tarsometatarsal joints with capsulotomies
(Heyman procedure). Medial release of the talocalcaneal joint.
Lengthening of the tendon Achilles." One week before the second
surgery, they removed the stitches from the first foot. After
manipulating my foot, they put me in a long leg plaster cast with
my knee flexed at 90 degrees. I wore that cast for three weeks, at
which time they put on a short leg cast. I mention this because
you can imagine how uncomfortable that was for a child. For a
period of time after the second surgery, both of my legs were
casted.

At Walter Reed, I remember looking out the window and
waiting for the activity director to come to the Children's Ward.
The children who could walk would push those of us who could
not walk in wheelchairs. Because they only operated on one foot
at a time, my hospital stay lasted 42 days. I was discharged at the
end of September.

Once the surgeries were done, I was still casted for a while.
The cast covered most of my leg for the first couple of weeks.
Then, I was put in short leg casts. I have a picture from a family
reunion that shows me sitting on my cousin's horse with the cast
on my foot. I could walk some. I remember having a rubber heel
on the bottom of my casts. My mom would put socks over the top
of the casts. However, I could not run and play like a normal
four-year-old.

After the casts were removed, I still had to wear a brace

between my feet when I slept at night. My mom kept the instructions for my "New Fillauer Night Splint." It was basically two shoes with a bar connecting them. The angle of the shoes could be adjusted. When I turned on my side, one foot would be up in the air. The brace was very uncomfortable to sleep in. Naturally, I complained. My mom would reassure me and help me to fall asleep. Children can be very strong though—I got through that difficult time. My mom was my caregiver, cheerleader, and a shoulder to cry on. Parental involvement in the healing process is so important.

Growing up was often very difficult for me. There were many doctor appointments. I was the youngest of three girls. My oldest sister is three years older than I. My middle sister is only a year older. My sisters still tell a story about taking me on a walk in our neighborhood when I had casts on my feet. I was in a wagon, and they left me down the street when they went home. When my mom asked where I was, they pretended that they did not have another sister.

My sisters remember that when relatives came to visit us, I would get a quarter. They would get a dime. I would get a teddy bear; they would get nothing. (Probably because I was given the bear in the hospital when they were not there.) It's funny, I do not remember these stories—but they both say the same thing. I bring this up because as a child with clubfoot, I also had to deal with my sisters being jealous of the attention I received. Trust me, I would have been happy not to have the attention for that reason. As I mentioned earlier, I was in the hospital for 42 days. Because my father was still in the Army and had to report for duty, and my mother had two other children at home, I was often alone at the hospital. My father's brother moved to the area to help some. Clearly, my sisters did not understand what I was going through.

Buying shoes brought many tears. From a young age, I wanted to be able to wear the stylish saddle shoes that the other kids wore to school back in the 1960s. I had to wear high-top white "baby" shoes to first grade. I was so excited to finally be going to school with my older sisters. However, the other children made fun of my shoes. As we all know, children can be brutally honest and cruel at times. Besides needing support, my feet were very wide. Wide shoes were not as available then as they are now. Any time that I got new shoes, I had to have adjustments made. Every shoe had to have an "inner heel wedge, regular Thomas Heel, and molded leather sole cookies."

In May 1974 when I was 14, I wrote in my diary that, "I argued with mom and dad over Dr. Scholls sandals. Everyone is wearing them and I want a pair too. They are afraid that they will hurt my feet. I just want shoes I like." At one point in time, the doctor told my mom that I would need surgery again to lengthen my Achilles tendon. However, the doctor gave me some exercises to do. I remember standing on a step and stretching my heels downward. I had to do several repetitions. Apparently, it worked because I did not have to have surgery again. In June 1976, one diary entry says that I "went to foot doctor. He said that I don't have to go anymore." I was 16 years old when I no longer had to have regular yearly appointments with the foot doctor.

Shopping for shoes has never been something that I take lightly. It is much easier to find wide shoes now that I am older and wide shoes are more popular. However, my shoes have always cost more than the average person spends on shoes. As I became an adult, I was able to get stylish shoes because the shoe industry began offering more stylish shoes in wide. I have never been able to wear shoes from the less expensive shoe stores.

As an adult, I asked my mother why there were not any pictures of me as an infant with my feet showing. She said that having a baby with clubfoot was devasting for her and my father. They felt somehow responsible. That seems to be a common theme among parents when their children have some sort of issue. There was nothing they could have done to prevent my clubfeet. I know that. I have also been told that clubfoot can run in families.

My father told me that my paternal grandmother had some degree of clubfoot. (I do not remember her. She died of a heart attack when I was very young.) When my daughter was born, she had metatarsus adductus in one foot. This is where the foot is turned inward. She was casted for three months as an infant, which corrected her issue.

My daughter was born in Germany while my husband and I were stationed there. When people looked at my three-month-old infant with a cast on her foot, I felt like they were wondering what I had done to my child. It helped me to understand how my parents felt. Life seemed to come full circle when my mom was visiting in Germany and she helped me soak the cast off of my daughter's foot. The doctor did not want to cut it off. We soaked it in vinegar water and peeled it off. My mom had to do the same for me before each doctor appointment years prior. It took quite a while to do this. When I got older, they were able cut the casts off. I did get to see one of my casts as my mother saved it for many years.

When I tell people that I had clubfeet, they are surprised. By looking at me, you would never know. Other than the faint scars across the top of my feet, I have no visible signs. I have always wanted to share my story in hopes that it would inspire someone else. Yes, there were difficult times. However, I was a very active child once my feet were corrected. In high school, I skated four or five times a week at a roller-skating rink. I took skating lessons. I was a jogger. I was able to do anything that I wanted to do. I am now 63 years old. I walk my dogs a couple of miles a day on a regular basis. In September of last year, my husband and I biked 216 miles in six days from Buffalo to Syracuse, New York, along the Erie Canalway Trail. I lead a very active life.

That being said, I do have difficulty with my feet as a result of the surgeries. For the past 10 years or so, my feet have bothered me from time to time. I was fitted with orthotics that were made for my feet. I now have severe arthritis, primarily in my left foot. My doctor said that it was caused by the trauma of the surgery. For my entire life, I have had a sensitivity on the tops of my feet. To this day, if I accidentally hit the top of my feet on anything, the pain is excruciating. Luckily it only lasts a couple of minutes. I assume this is from the scar tissue.

As a child, I felt somewhat isolated and different. I did not know anyone else who had clubfoot when they were born. Most people did not even understand what that meant. As an adult, I feel thankful for the doctors and the team that were able to allow me to walk normally. I remember my mother mentioning one doctor in particular. In 2007, I was able to write to Dr. P. I found his information on the internet. It had always been my desire to thank the medical professionals. I was delighted to receive a letter back from him. However, he told me that he was not actually the one who performed the surgeries. My mom passed away in 2016. At that time, I got possession of all my medical records. I have copies of the notes from the Army. I found the names of the doctors who performed the surgeries. Recently I sent each of them a letter. I feel very blessed to have had the care that was given to me. There are many children in countries around the world who are not as fortunate.

My advice to parents of children born with clubfoot: your child will be okay. Don't blame yourself. There is no way that you could have prevented it. Clubfoot can be corrected. Advancements have been made. With the Ponseti method, very few children need to have surgery. Healing doesn't happen overnight. It is a process that you will need to help your child through. Take pictures. Your children will want to know what their feet looked like. Share your story so that others can be encouraged. Reach out to others. Ask your doctor if there are other parents that they can give your information to so that you can connect and support each other. I also found a Facebook group that supports parents and children who have been affected by clubfoot.

Lastly, look for organizations where you can give back. This past year, I became aware of a nonprofit organization called Hope Walks that helps kids in low-income countries get quality club-foot care using the Ponseti method. Hope Walks even provides braces to children in Ethiopia where I was born! They provide supplies for painting parties to paint the leathers that are attached to the braces. They have found that the children love having colorful shoes. They are more apt to wear the necessary brace. I attended a painting party and held a couple of painting parties with friends from my church. My oldest sister teaches nursing. I shared my story with her students and then led them in painting the leathers. Training the next generation is very important. Her students are now aware of clubfeet. My hope is that hearing my story will help them when they come across a child with a deformity.

I am very thankful to God for the experiences that I have had in my life. Would I have chosen to have clubfeet? Of course not. However, it is part of who I am. I have always had a sense of grati-tude that I do not walk with a limp or other visible sign. I feel extremely blessed to be able to share my story and impact the lives of others.

who would have thought?

Christopher Myers

WHO WOULD HAVE THOUGHT that I, the first child of a Physical Education teacher mother and her Marine Corps Major husband would be born with two clubbed feet? There are no rules, there is no pattern, stereotypes don't matter, and it's nobody's fault! It just happens. At 9:07 on Sunday morning, March 28, 1965, in Oceanside, California, I came into the world.

Earlier that spring, I was bumping around inside my mom as she rode her horse, Mountain Bounty. Believe it or not, I still mimic the bumpity, bumpity, bumpity of the horse's canter as I often rock myself to sleep. The farm where Mom rode was just below Mission San Luis Rey where I was to be christened. The colors of the chapel are vivid to me still all these years later and I'm convinced they influenced my choosing to go to art school.

As the doctor held me, not much was said: I looked like a baby flamingo with two swollen pink legs and unusual feet rather than a baby boy. I can only imagine the emotions at that moment as my new mother, father, and grandparents stared.

Who would have thought that, at that moment in the hospital, the leading pediatric podiatrist from Newark, New Jersey, was visiting? Dr. Sharp had my leg and feet in casts before we went home.

Burdened with a tough reality, my mother placed me on her bed and prayed, "Lord, please help me." It was more than the weekly cast removal and replacement that weighed heavy on her heart. I think the enjoyment of a child with a disability right out of the gate can be strained. Mom not only wanted to be a good mother and do what was necessary for my healing, but also wanted to enjoy me as a healthy baby.

Like experiencing the horse rides when I was in Mom's body and looking up and being affected by the colors in the chapel during my christening, early experiences were fundamental building blocks to my character.

"You were always chatty with strangers as I held you," my mother recalls. She brought me with her to school as she led gymnastics practice. "The students loved you. And you'd be right there asking them questions and making them laugh. The braces didn't stop you."

Obstacles to overcome have made me stronger, like when my mother flew with me to Newark, New Jersey, for surgery as the riots of 1967 were in full swing. Dr. Sharp had determined that my left Achilles tendon needed surgery to provide a better range of motion. Outfitted with the new cast, I was unbalanced as I walked around the pool where we stayed, and you can guess what happened. Pomolly, a St. Bernard, barked wildly and ensured my safety as adults swiftly came to my rescue. Despite the unexpected plunge into the pool, I've never tired of swimming out into the ocean or playing endlessly in pools.

Who would have thought that, after all the stretching, brace wearing, and shoes that didn't fit my feet properly, I'd be the fastest kid in school in sixth grade? Or who would have imagined I'd be on swim team, or starting defensive player in soccer and lacrosse in high school? Even with a left foot a size and a half smaller than the right foot!

Growing up, my parents seldom talked about my clubbed feet. They agreed early on that they didn't want me to identify with my deformity, nor allow it to define me. I'm glad about that! It hasn't defined me, and who I am as a result of solid coaching by loving parents and those around me is miraculous. I've been made stronger by a deformity, because I saw the power of healing.

I've become involved in an organization, Hope Walks, that supports clubfoot clinics around the world. I never thought to reach out and get involved until one day while on the beach here in St. Augustine, Florida, I watched a young boy hobble across the sand with clubbed feet that had gone untreated. I sobbed with recognition that I could have been that boy. And at that moment, it hit me—God had answered my mom's prayer. I'm proof of it and, like her, I've asked God to help me help others.

Who would have thought that nearly six decades since that Sunday morning in Oceanside, not only is my deformity healed, but my identity is, too? Lots of people said hurtful words about my feet and the way I walked as I grew up. Emotional scars are far worse than the scar on my left ankle. I continue to forgive others for their ignorance, and I continue to forgive myself when I see my limitations.

I've learned that the miracle of healing doesn't always happen overnight. Healing is a robust word, because it represents the physical, emotional, and spiritual. As I've grown up with club-foot, learned about orthotics, and taken care as I travel, I'm grateful because the choices I've made and challenges that I've overcome have given me a rich library of how I got to be me. I become better as the healing continues every day.

The healing process makes us all better! If you have clubbed feet or if you are a parent, caregiver, friend, or relative of someone with clubfoot, remain open to how the healing process unfolds. And remember, we're not in this alone. Just ask, "Lord, please help me." You'll be amazed at the outcome!

you've got this

a poem for clubfoot parents
Katherine Kiedaisch

"It's treatable," they tell you
On 20-week ultrasound day.
Confusion and guilt rush in—
"Clubfoot is not your fault," they say.

After some frantic home research
Seeing photos of tiny, crooked feet,
You were never expecting this;
It's too difficult to believe.

At first, you're fearful and full of nerves,
But then you change your tone.
After joining social media groups,
You don't feel quite so alone.

Before long, the big day comes:
You finally meet your baby boy.
His precious face melts your heart.
Fear fades, and all you feel is joy!

Katherine Kiedaisch

His tiny, twisted feet
Are perfect in your eyes.
You'll move mountains to protect him,
To soothe his gentle cries.

Those first few days are fleeting,
A blur of bare toes and soft skin,
Certainly not enough time
To get all of your kisses in.

Treatments begin, the stress is real;
His appointments are so far away.
Weekly casting, painful, heavy legs,
And "Don't forget, no footie PJs!"

Strangers stare, they ask rude questions,
They think that he is broken.
But they don't know his story.
It's just beginning, and unspoken.

You make it work, you figure it out;
Treatments stop feeling so strange.
With each new cast, and the tenotomy,
You can already see a huge change.

And when it's time for boots and bar,
Though it's nothing you can't handle,
Who would have thought such loss of sleep
Could come from two little sandals?

Your boy turns one, and soon, you're done
With the blisters of 23-hour wear.
He's crawling now, and suddenly—Wow!
He's trying to climb the stairs!

Soon, he's walking and he's talking.
Once crooked feet, now nice and straight.
Nighttime is easy, toddler daycare is fun.
He's loving life and doing great!

Don't forget, he'll never remember
The tears and pain from back then.
His fifth birthday is here. It's time to cheer—
You've made it to the end!

You never thought you'd come this far,
Or get to see the day
When your little clubfoot cutie
Gets to dance and jump and play.

Now every time you watch him run
Or amaze you with skills anew,
Just remember where you started,
And how clubfoot couldn't beat you.

acknowledgments

From Betsy:

Thank you, Nicole Bytnerowicz and Jill Harold, for your enthusiastic support for this project when it was in the idea stage.

Maureen, you're amazing—it was wonderful to work with you. Lita Kurth, your insights and advice about developing this anthology are much appreciated. Anthony Francis, Kate Luce, and Tessa Miller, thank you for reading an early version of this book and giving feedback.

From Maureen:

I would like to thank my husband, Brian, for his continued belief in my mission to help clubfoot parents share their voices. To my older two girls for being the best sisters to their own clubfoot sister. To my clubfoot superstar, you are my eternal inspiration. Thank you for choosing me to be your mom. You never cease to amaze me.

To Betsy, thank you for allowing me to be a part of this project. I am so grateful that our paths converged and for your consistent support of clubfoot parents everywhere.

From both of us:

To all the clubfoot parents who submitted a piece for this anthology, your contributions are everything and your story will impact so many lives. And to clubfoot parents everywhere, you are the inspiration for it all.

To the Thinking Ink Press team, thank you for believing in this book and making it happen. Special thanks to Liza Olmsted for her editing and formatting expertise, to Keiko O'Leary for poetry editing, and to Marilyn Horn for her copy editing.

about the editors

Betsy Miller

Betsy Miller is the author of *The Parents' Guide to Clubfoot* and *Beyond Boots 'n' Bars: A Journal for Clubfoot Parents* and coauthor of *Hip, Hop, Hooray for Brooklynn!*, a picture book about a bunny with clubfoot. She cofounded Thinking Ink Press, a small publisher based in Silicon Valley.

When she's not writing, editing, or publishing, Betsy enjoys taking nature walks, traveling, and reading. She lives in Northern California with her husband.

Maureen Hoff

Maureen Hoff is the author of *Clubfoot Chronicles* and host of *A Clubfoot Mom* podcast. She is the mother to three girls, the youngest of whom was born with bilateral clubfoot. Maureen works to help other parents navigate their child's clubfoot journey and believes strongly in sharing the voices of all clubfoot community members.

Maureen currently lives in Colorado with her husband and children. You can contact her at MaureenHoff.com.

Also by Betsy Miller

- *The Parents' Guide to Clubfoot*
- *Beyond Boots 'n' Bars: A Journal for Clubfoot Parents*
- *Hip, Hop, Hooray for Brooklynn!* children's picture book by Jill Harold and Betsy Miller
- *Bunny Fun Coloring Book for Kids: Let's Play!* by Jill Harold and Betsy Miller

Also by Maureen Hoff

- *Clubfoot Chronicles: Tips for Helping Your Clubfoot Cutie During Treatment*
- *A Clubfoot Mom* podcast
- "Understanding Clubfoot Treatment" on-demand class, BabySparks.com

Also by Chloe Howard

- *Stand Beautiful: A story of brokenness, beauty and embracing it all*
- *Stand Beautiful* children's picture book
- "How I redefined my labels and left my bully behind" TEDx Santa Barbara talk, 2016

More Clubfoot Picture Books

- *Boots & Barnyard Boogie* by Rachel Reinsch
- *My Big Boots* by Dr. Mitzi Williams with Dr. Matthew Dobbs and Dr. Scott Kaiser
- *My Clever Night-Night Shoes* by Karen Mara Moss
- *One in 1000* by Sonia Alcon
- *Pete's Neat Feet* by Damaris Gibson

Other Clubfoot Resources and Organizations

- **26th Avenue Clubfoot Essentials** (custom clubfoot boots and bar covers): 26thAveClubfoot-Essentials.com
- **Canadian Clubfoot Support Society**: Clubfoot.ca
- **Clubfoot CARES**: ClubfootCARES.org
- **Clubfoot Hub**: ClubfootHub.com
- **Global Clubfoot Initiative**: GlobalClubfoot.com
- **No Surgery 4 Clubfoot**: NoSurgery4Clubfoot.com
- **Ponseti International Association**: Ponseti.info
- **STEPS Clubfoot Care**: STEPS.org.za
- **STEPS Worldwide**: STEPSWorldwide.org

Connect with the Editors and Authors

Betsy Miller
Email: betsy@thinkinginkpress.com

Maureen Hoff
Website: MaureenHoff.com

Laura (Rayl) Bucknam
Dillsburg, PA
Facebook: Laura-Mike Bucknam

Aaron and Ann-Jeanette England
Instagram: @englandcalifornia

Chloe Howard
Instagram: @itschloehoward
Website: StandBeautiful.me

Lori T. Howard
Website: LoriTHoward.com

Katherine Kiedaisch
Email: katherinekiedaisch@gmail.com

Delphine Le Roux
Instagram: @delphine_lrx

Casey Murphy
Email: caseyannemurphy@gmail.com

Christopher Myers
Website: ChristopherMichaelMyers.com

Jessica Norris
Email: jessicanorris417@gmail.com
Instagram: @jessica.n.norris

Chidiogo Obiesie
LinkedIn: Chidiogo Obiesie

Jennifer L. Perrotta
Email: jenn1seven@yahoo.com

About Thinking Ink Press

Thinking Ink Press has been publishing books for kids and adults about children's health topics, including clubfoot, since 2015. We are a small book publishing company run by four authors with a love for the printed word. We publish traditional books in several genres, as well as innovative formats including hand-folded books and literary postcards.

Our Books about Clubfoot

Picture book: *Hip, Hop, Hooray for Brooklynn!*
by Jill Harold & Betsy Miller

Bunny Fun Coloring Book for Kids: Let's Play!
by Jill Harold & Betsy Miller

Beyond Boots 'n' Bars: A Journal for Clubfoot Parents by Betsy Miller

Clubfoot Mailing List

Get clubfoot news and resources by email, starting with free coloring book pages.
Visit **ThinkingInkPress.com/clubfoot**.

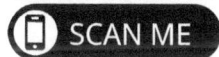

SCAN ME